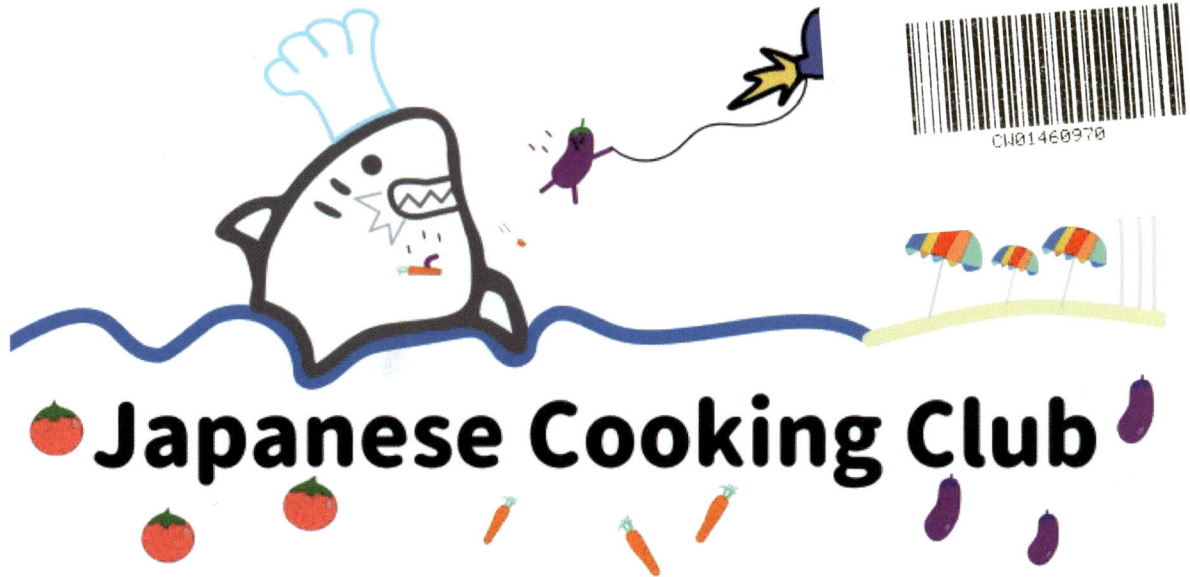

Japanese Cooking Club

Getting started with

plant-based Japanese foods

by Pat Tokuyama

For free video training and resources to help you cook plant-based Japanese food, visit alldayieat.com/go/bookresources

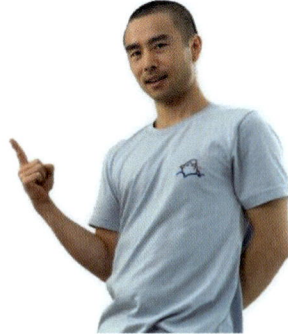

For recipes, books, and other products visit www.alldayieat.com

all day i eat like a shark LLC

3857 Birch St. #23

Newport Beach, CA 92660

ISBN 978-1-7328907-1-8 (Print)

Who this cookbook is for

- **You're ready to take responsibility for the food you eat so you can live a healthier and longer life**
- **You want to incorporate more vegetables and healthier cooking into your lifestyle**
- **You enjoy cooking plant-based food and you're looking for something new**
- **You're looking for a new way to enjoy Japanese food**
- **You know nothing about plant-based food or Japanese food and are ready to learn**

Anyone can learn to cook delicious, plant-based Japanese food.

Whether you're a complete newbie to cooking or have a decent amount of experience in the kitchen, the recipes in this book will give you a solid foundation in plant-based Japanese cuisine.

This cookbook contains many of the recipes I've shared with the Japanese Cooking Club members over the past year. And as many of our members have found, this type of cooking can be easier (and even more delicious) than you might think!

Many of these dishes are simple to make and yet, as refined as you would expect traditional Japanese food to be. They not only offer the many health benefits of a plant-based diet, but also rich Japanese flavors, textures, and aromas that'll have you and your loved ones asking for more.

And if you enjoy cooking and eating as much as the Club members and me, this could be the very beginning of a tasty, lifelong, plant-based journey. And chances are, you're gonna love what lies ahead.

From here on out, you can use your new knowledge to continue your explorations as you delve deeper into the delicious world of Japanese cuisine.

Plus - a lot of what you'll learn here can also be applied to other cuisines both plant-based and non-plant-based cooking. When using this book, consider how you can apply aspects of these recipes to other types of cooking.

And expect *more* magic to happen in your kitchen *more* often!

Ikagadeshouka?（いかがでしょうか How's that sound?）

-Pat

Contents

From pharmacist to plant-based cooking advocate

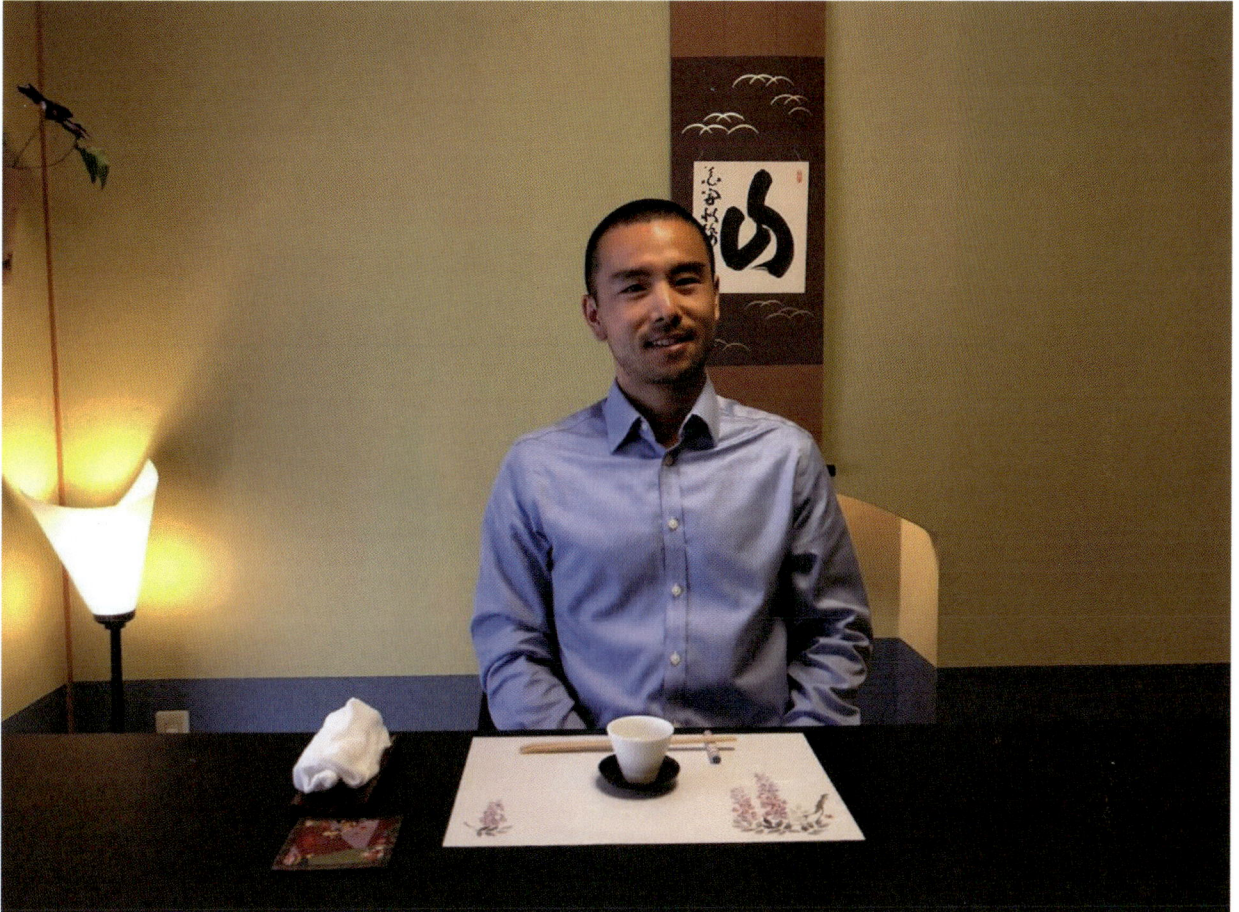

Konnichiwa! (こんにちは - Hello)

If we haven't met before, I'm Pat Tokuyama, Pharm.D., BCPS, a pharmacist by training and founder of the Japanese Cooking Club.

Thank you for joining me on this journey and taking the first of many baby steps toward making plant-based Japanese food a part of your life.

I became a pharmacist so I could help people using my knowledge of medicine. Ironically, I now leverage my knowledge to help people stay off and reduce their reliance on medicines by advocating plant-based Japanese food.

The gap in healthcare

After working almost two decades in the healthcare industry, I've come to realize one of the biggest gaps in healthcare today remains largely ignored: diet (the food you eat) and exercise.

While working in a clinic, I cared for many sick patients first hand, and rounded with the medical team while working in the hospital. Often times, these patients were admitted for complications of heart disease, diabetes, and or obesity. From reading their medical charts, it was clear that their poor health condition could have been prevented.

Of course, some people may never develop conditions despite unhealthy habits.

But for many of us, our lifestyle habits like regular exercise and the food we eat and can make a meaningful difference to our health. And especially so, as we get older.

Today, diabetes and heart disease medications are some of the highest contributors to health plan drug costs, especially in the Medicare population (those aged 65 years or older). In order to reverse that trend, something needs to change.

And that change starts with us.

Making health a priority

We need to make our health a priority, by being more mindful of the foods we eat and the quality and quantity of exercise we do.

Although the importance of diet and exercise is clearly documented in our national treatment guidelines for many chronic diseases, it's not emphasized enough.

It's true - it's easier to swallow a pill than change your habits.

But I believe with a more mindful way of living - as it pertains to food you eat and exercise - you can prevent certain chronic diseases from occurring in the first place.

In medicine, this is called primary prevention: stopping the disease from happening in the first place.

And no, it's never too late.

My mission

A few years ago I set myself a goal to never have to take prescription medications for chronic diseases like high blood pressure, high cholesterol or diabetes.

Having significant family history of cancer, diabetes, and heart disease, it's a goal I set out to accomplish each day.

To give you some perspective, my dad takes more than 7 chronic medications and last year had a stent placed to open one of his clogged heart arteries. I don't want to be in that place when I'm older and I don't want you to be either.

I've made it my mission to empower you so you can also make healthy food choices for you and your loved ones with plant-based Japanese food.

Through this book and my online training programs, I want to close the gap in healthcare by stressing the importance of cooking plant-based foods so that you can live a longer and healthier life.

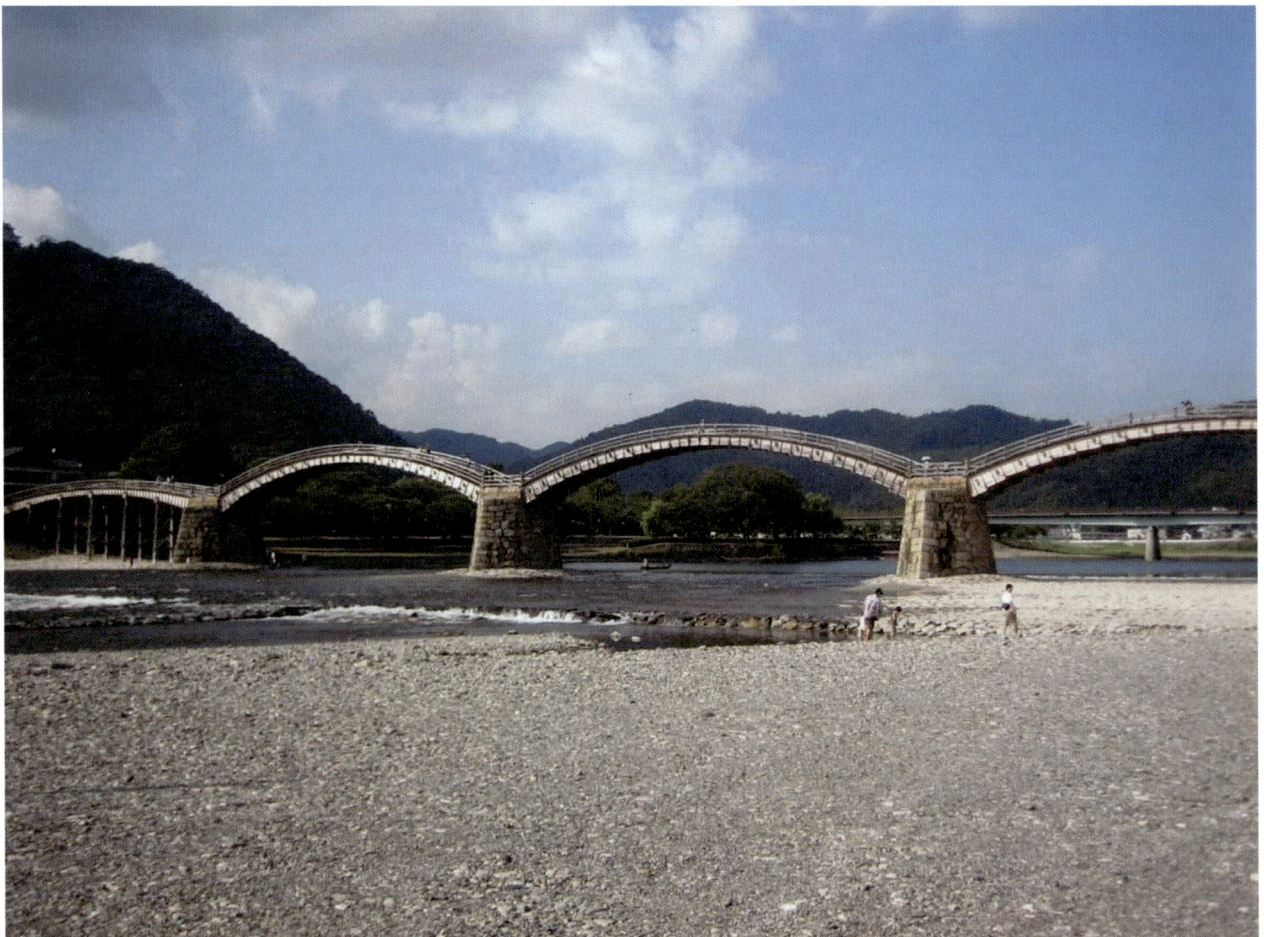

Kintaikyo Bridge, Iwakuni, Japan

Making plant-based foods part of your life

So... you might be wondering, how do you start to incorporate plant-based food into your life?

Well, that depends on you and your unique situation. Everyone's on a different path with their own individual needs, expectations, and goals.

What I can share are several things that will help you along the way:

- taking it step by step
- giving yourself credit for each step you make
- enjoying the process

It may not be easy to change old habits. Do what you can and take baby steps because every dish and every effort counts.

Wherever you are, it's progress that matters, not perfection. Those small incremental changes all add up, especially in the long run.

It might even be useful to keep track of your progress by writing it down so you can see how much progress you've made over time.

Remember, we all started somewhere. And you're right where you need to be right now. Ignore what other people are doing and don't compare yourself to them.

Everyone has different needs and wants and starts in a different place.

Where ever you are in life there'll always be someone in ahead of you and behind you.

Keep your head down and focus on your needs. Take note of where you're starting today and where you're going tomorrow.

That's all that matters.

As long as you're making little improvements and making plant-based foods a more regular part of your lifestyle, eventually it'll become second nature to you.

And with that positive reinforcement and being kind to yourself, you'll get to where you want to go. It's not a matter of *if you'll get there*, but when.

I wish you the best in your cooking adventures and invite you to join our community.

Plant-based Japanese Cooking Made Simple Community

Connecting with other like-minded home cooks will help you grow and stay committed to cooking and eating healthier with plant-based Japanese food!

Request access at alldayieat.com/go/community

Douzo yoroshiku onegaiitashimasu

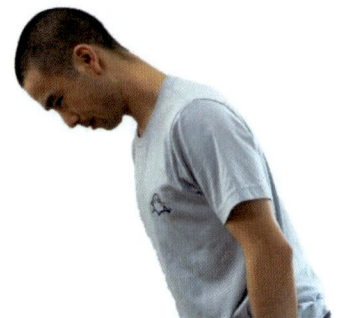

(どうぞよろしくお願いいたします let's be good to each other)

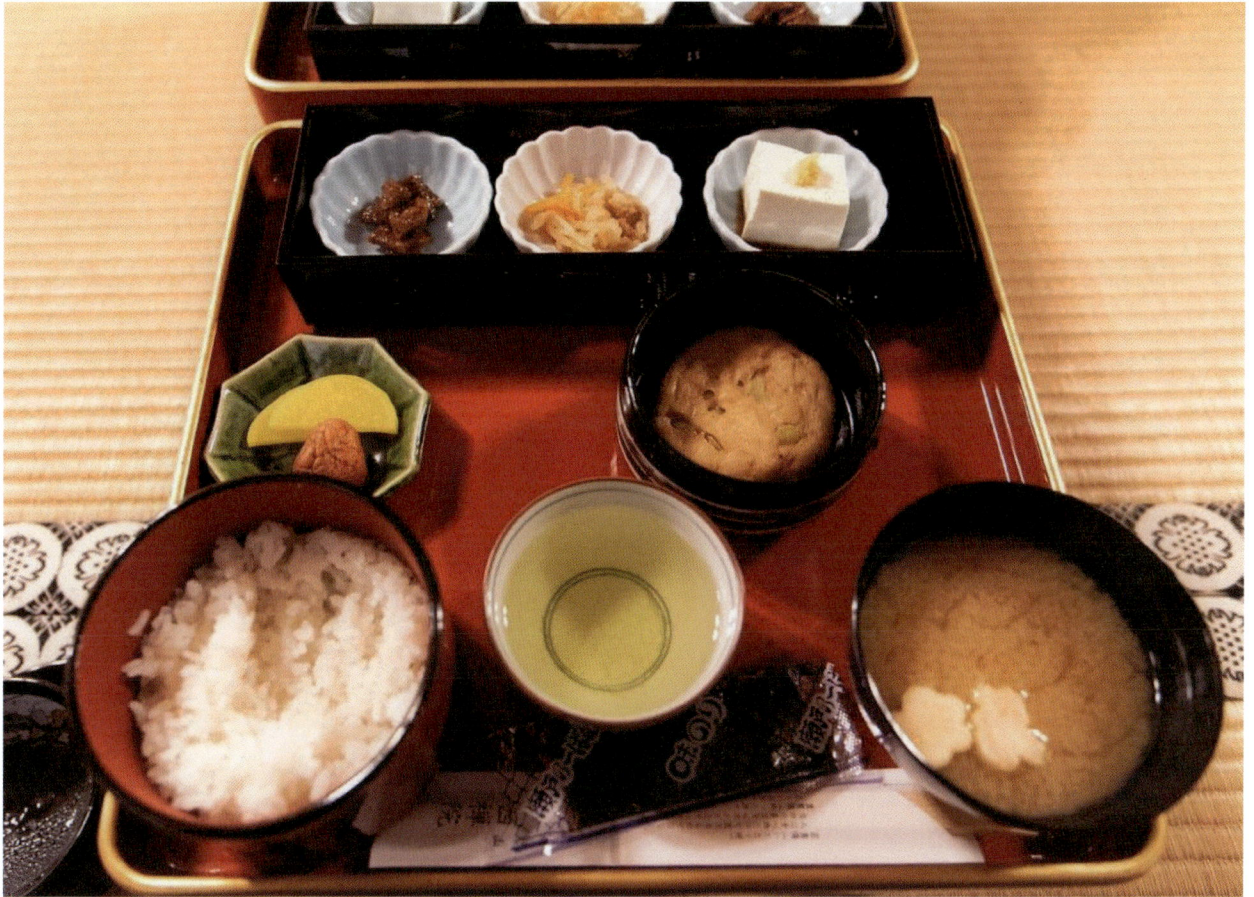

Shojin Ryouri breakfast, Mount Koya, Japan

What is a 'plant-based' diet?

The whole food plant-based (WFPB) diet is something that I learned about several years ago by accident.

If you've never heard of the whole food plant-based diet, in short the goal is to eat foods that consist of plants (fruits, vegetables, beans, legumes, grains etc) as close to their natural states as possible. This also means minimal use of processed or refined foods.

The whole food plant-based diet is different from other 'diets' in that it places emphasis on including these ingredients rather than exclusion.

It's a different way of eating, not 'diet' as in a structured meal plan you try for a short while and then give up on.

Some people confuse vegan and plant-based diets as equivalent and use them interchangeably in conversations but they are fundamentally different.

Vegans exclude all animal products and the reason behind it may have more to do with ethics rather than health.

The plant-based food lifestyle is about health first and foremost and incorporating as much whole plant foods into each meal as you can. That's what the plant-based diet is at its core.

It's not vegan or vegetarian.

It's unique in its own way.

Health benefits

Whole food plant-based foods have been linked to many health benefits, such as preventing heart disease, diabetes, cancer, obesity and other chronic diseases. As someone who works in healthcare and has significant family history of chronic disease, you can see why it appeals to me.

Plant-based foods seem to have grown in popularity recently for that reason, which is good and a step in the right direction.

As plant-based foods become more common, people may associate anything 'plant-based' as healthy. However, the key thing to remember is that it's whole food plant-based foods that have been shown to provide health benefits in clinical trials.

Can you eat other foods?

For those who are strict and follow the whole food plant-based diet to the letter, this means no oils, sugar, syrup, flour, white rice or other refined products.

However, my philosophy is and always has been to follow the spirit of whole food plant-based without completely giving up other things I love.

I confess I love eating white rice... and spicy extra-virgin olive oil... and some sweets on occasion...

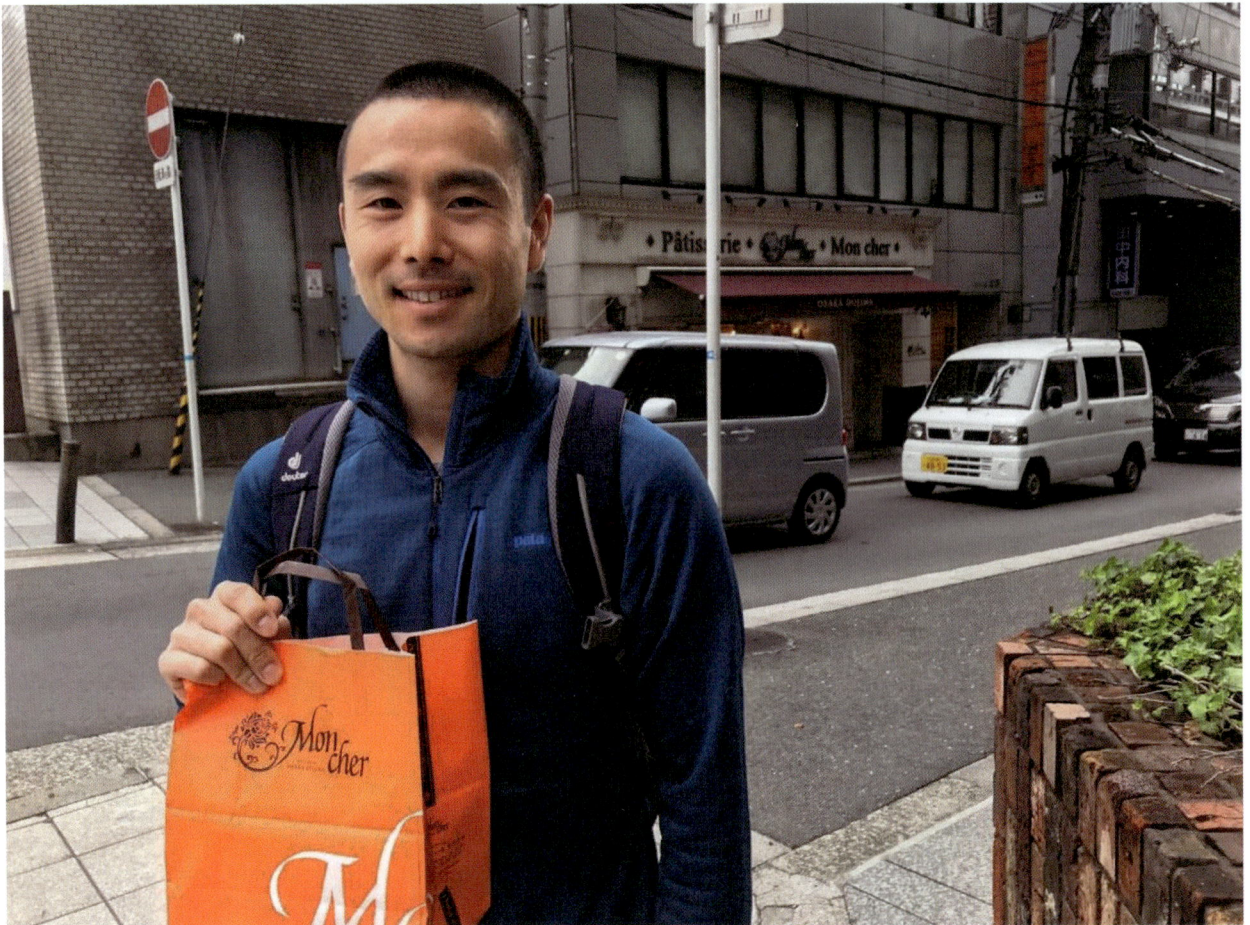
Mon-cher Patiesserie, Osaka, Japan

For me, life just wouldn't be as fulfilling.

I believe a healthy lifestyle allows you to enjoy what you want in moderation, without feeling shameful or guilty.

And if you do cut back on your consumption of meat or seafood, when you do have it, it might be for a special occasion (like celebrating a birthday, anniversary, or in tribute to your past life).

So yes. You can eat other foods.

And I'd encourage you to do so in moderation, especially if you're just starting out. It might make the transition easier for you (remember, baby steps!) You know what's right for you and your family.

The point of the whole-food plant-based diet is to maximize whole plant foods as much as you can. By doing this, over time you may find that you have less and less cravings for non plant-based foods anyway.

What can Japanese cuisine offer?

In the spirit of whole food plant-based lifestyle, you'll find most of the dishes in this book are congruent with the main aspects of a whole food plant-based diet.

This means that this cookbook emphasizes Japanese foods made from whole foods. Plant foods with naturally produced Japanese seasonings and minimally processed foods/ingredients.

Yes, Japanese food can and does call for a lot of fish and fish products.

And yes, it's quite simple to avoid using them... if that's a goal of yours.

If you're skeptical, perhaps this cookbook will give you a new perspective.

And if you're anything like the cooking club members and me, you may notice your palate may begin to change and those non plant-based food cravings will begin to subside and even go away completely.

There's nothing like eating a clean, plant-based meal!

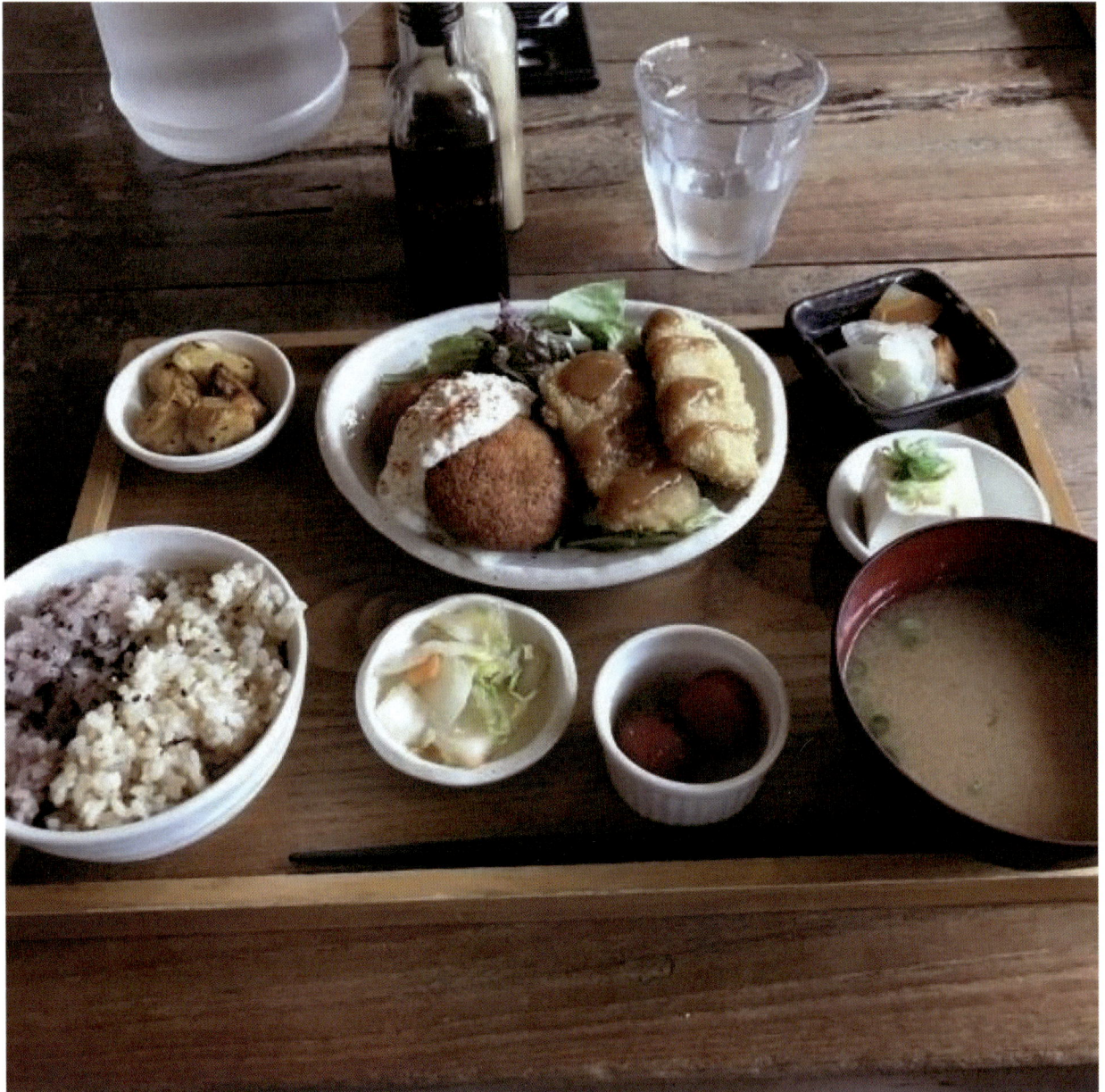

Plant-based lunch, Mumokuteki cafe, Kyoto, Japan

What is Japanese food?

If you're new to Japanese food and cooking, you might be wondering what real Japanese food is.

Well, first let's talk about what I mean by 'real'. When I say 'real' I'm referring to the type of food you'll find if you visit Japan. So what type of food will you find in Japan?

Like many modern countries, it can be extremely diverse. Especially if you're talking about some of the biggest cities like Tokyo or Osaka.

Walking around you'll discover a wide variety of restaurants and different cuisines, ranging from traditional (和食 washoku) to Western, Asian, African and everything else in between.

Japanese food (outside of Japan) usually seems to consist of something like sushi, ramen and beef bowls, or sweets like mochi and matcha ice cream.

And I get why... it tastes good!

But if you aren't too familiar with Japanese food, there's so much more just waiting for you to discover and enjoy.

Wafu (和風 Japanese-style)

Because of many outside influences on Japan over the last century, a lot has been adapted. These foreign foods have since been tailored and refined for the Japanese palate and incorporated into Japanese style home cooking.

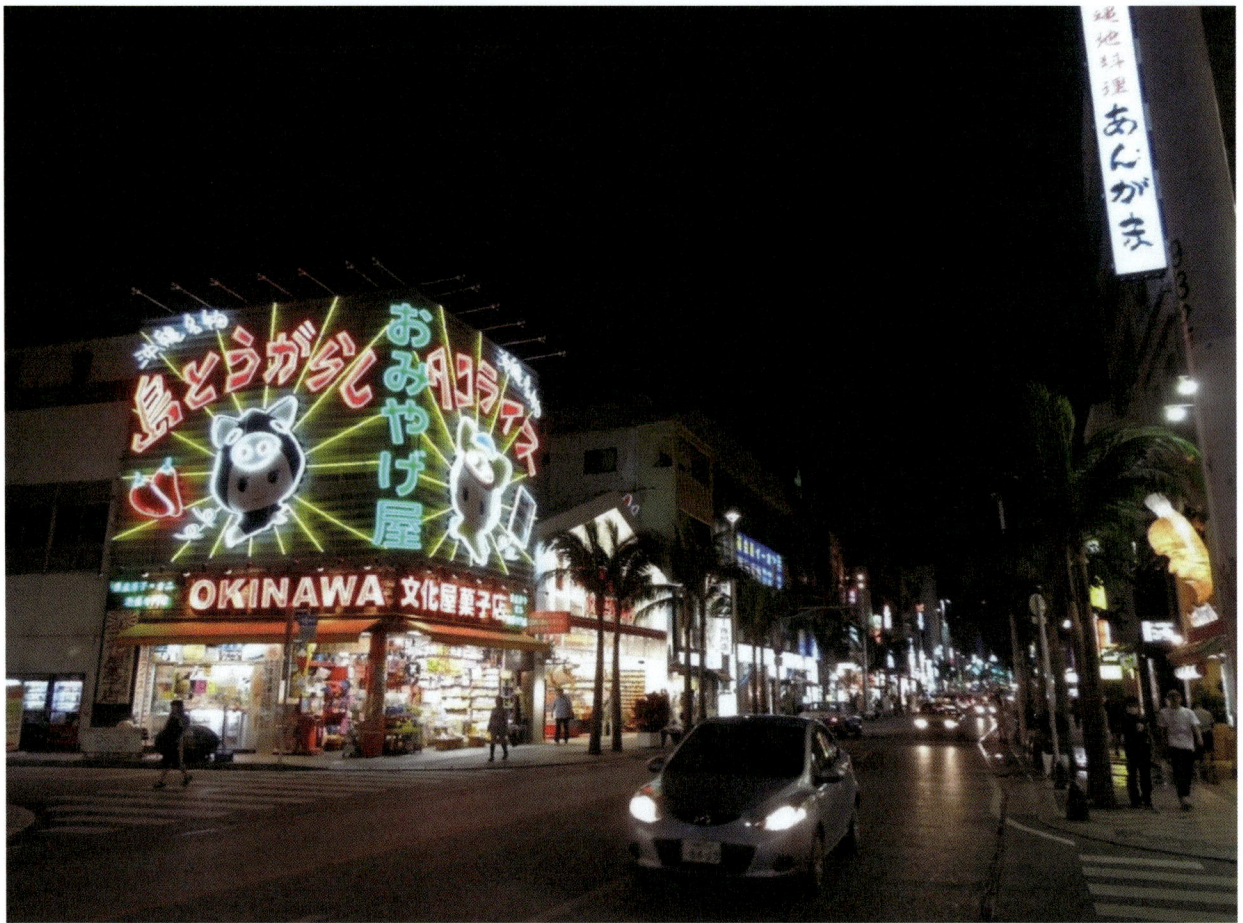
Kokusaidori in Naha, Okinawa

Some of my favorites include Japanese Italian food (especially pasta), Japanese French pastries and Japanese Indian curries.

These Japanese foods might not be initially the first thing you think of when you think of Japanese food. But for me, recreating these dishes in my kitchen very much reminds me of Japan and all the delicious food I ate while living in and traveling the country.

While you might think of these wafu foods, as fusion, which to some may be a dirty word. They're a bit better than fusion, at least that which I've experienced here in the US, but I could very well be biased. ;)

These wafu foods are very distinct and unique in their own style, often incorporating Japanese techniques, and of course ingredients.

Endless possibilities

And that's what makes 'real' Japanese food so very, very diverse!

Since you're reading this book, I hope you'll be happy to know that.

You'd be hard pressed to ever get bored with Japanese food.

You can easily eat and cook your way through an endless variety of Japanese foods from the comfort of your kitchen.

As you go through this cookbook, you'll discover a variety of traditional Japanese dishes that are simple, delicious, and easy to make.

Ready to get started?

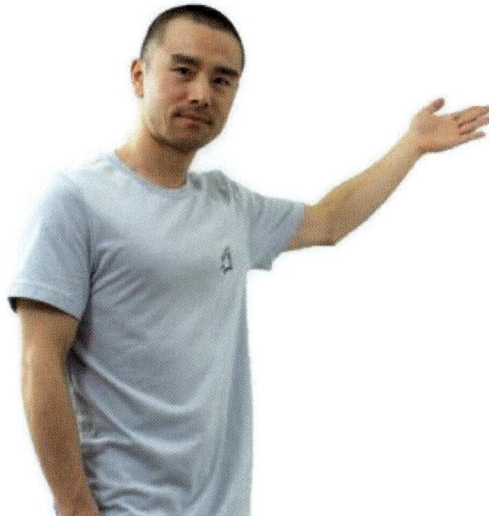

Ikuzo (行くぞ Let's go!)

Japanese tofu set meal

Japanese Pantry Shopping List

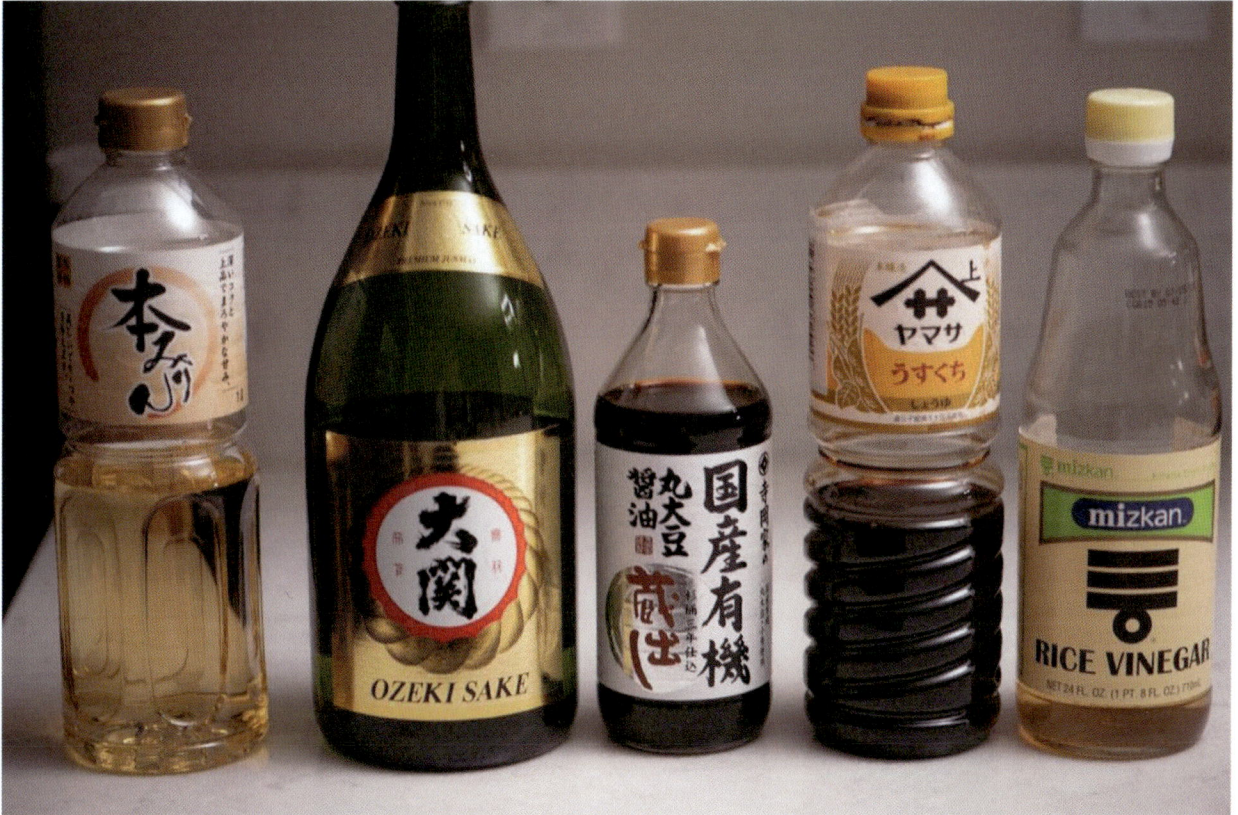

(Left to right) Hon-mirin, sake, soy sauce, light soy sauce, rice vinegar

Below is a basic list of Japanese ingredients you'll need for the recipes in this book.

Mirin (味醂 sweet sake)

There are two types of mirin: hon-mirin (本みりん true mirin) and aji-mirin (味み りん mirin flavor). Aji-mirin may be easier to find and will provide the same flavor as hon-mirin. You can use them interchangeably.

Osake (お酒 sake)

If you can, try to avoid cooking sake, because it has added salt which is not necessary. You don't need to buy a pricey drinking sake either, two brands I often use are Ozeki and Gekkeikan.

Shouyu (醤油 soy sauce)

Look for brands made in Japan such as Kikkoman. If you want Japanese flavors, do not substitute with a non-Japanese soy sauce.

There are five common types of soy sauce:

- Shouyu or koikuchi shouyu (濃口醤油 regular soy sauce)
- Usukuchi shouyu (薄口醤油 light soy sauce)
- Genen shouyu (減塩醤油 low-sodium soy sauce)
- Tamari (たまり the name for the liquid that pools during miso production)
- Saishikomi (再仕込み twice brewed soy sauce)

If you're just starting out, get a low-sodium soy sauce and a light soy sauce. These are the two most commonly used types of soy sauce in Japanese cuisine.

Osu (お酢 rice vinegar)

Rice vinegar is used to make shari (シャリ sushi rice), pickles, as a condiment for gyoza (餃子 potstickers), and many other things. It has a sharper taste than white wine vinegar and can be used in many of the same ways as

Western vinegars. If you can find kurozu (黒酢 black vinegar), that's a good way to change up the flavor slightly for dressings and other vinegar based seasonings. It's made from brown rice and has a darker color.

Gomaabura (胡麻油 sesame oil)

Sesame oil is a dark brown oil used mainly for flavor and aroma. You don't need much of it so a bottle will last you a while. There is also another type called taihaku gomaabura (太白胡麻油 white sesame oil). This oil is clear (like canola oil) and can also be used for baking because it has a much lighter flavor and aroma. It may be worth trying for a lighter sesame flavor in certain recipes such as salad dressings.

Dashi (だし stock/broth)

Dashi can be made from scratch using a variety of ingredients. For example, it can be made using katsuobushi (鰹節 dried, fermented fish flakes), niboshi (煮干し dried sardines), konbu (昆布 dried kelp) or shiitake (干し椎茸 dried shiitake mushrooms). These can be used alone or in combination, and with or without other vegetables and ingredients.

You'll learn how to make dashi from scratch on page 30. If you don't want to make it from scratch, you can purchase ready-to-use dashi in the form of dashi powder or dashi packs, which work in the same way as a tea bag.

Make sure to check the ingredients of ready-to-use dashi so you know what's in it. Some brands add salt and or MSG to it. You can find examples of brands I like that use minimal additives at alldayieat.com/go/bookresources.

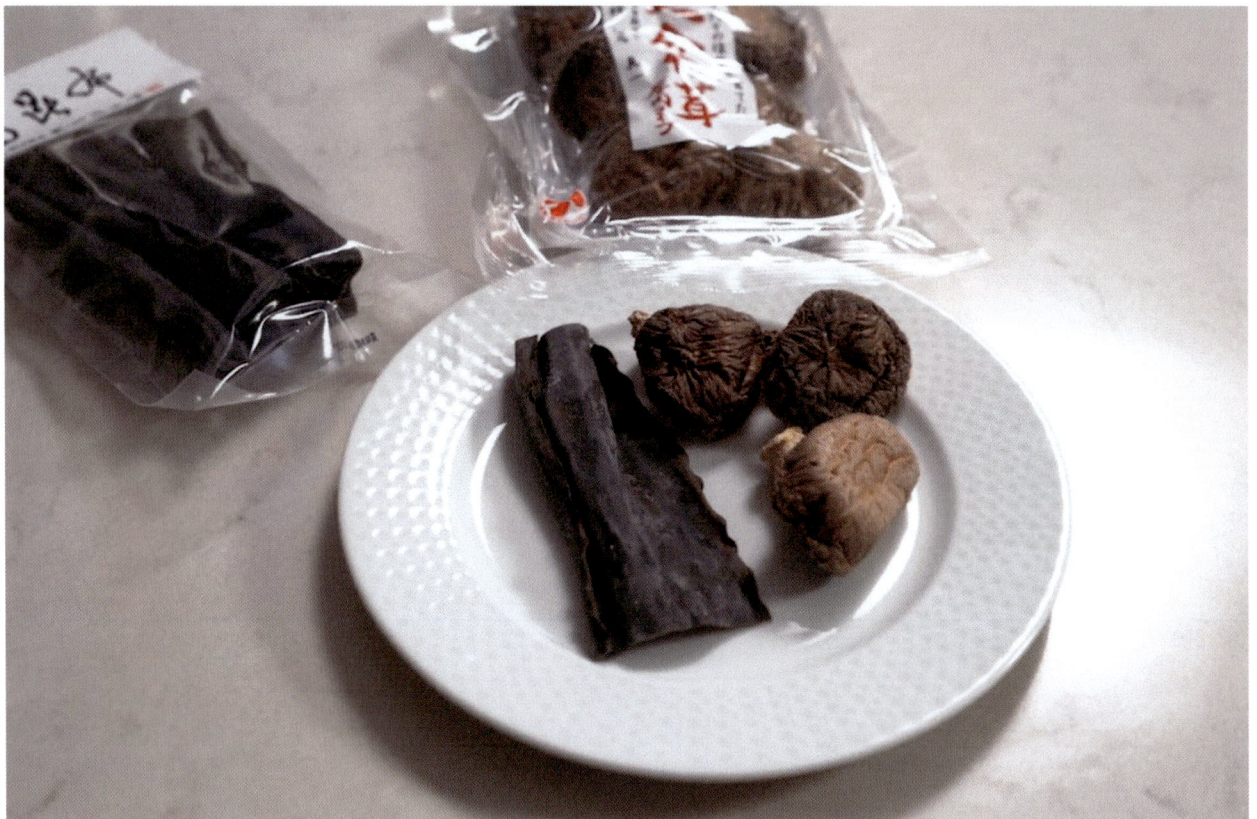

Dried konbu and dried shiitake mushrooms

Miso 味噌

Two of the most common types are akamiso (赤味噌 red miso) and shiromiso (白味噌 white miso). While they can be used interchangeably for soup, white is sweeter and less strong in flavor so works better as a marinade and in sauces.

I prefer akamiso in soup. You can also mix different miso pastes to make a unique flavor if you want to try something different.

Be mindful that some miso pastes contain dashi and so are intended to be used in soups. You may want to double check the ingredients on the label.

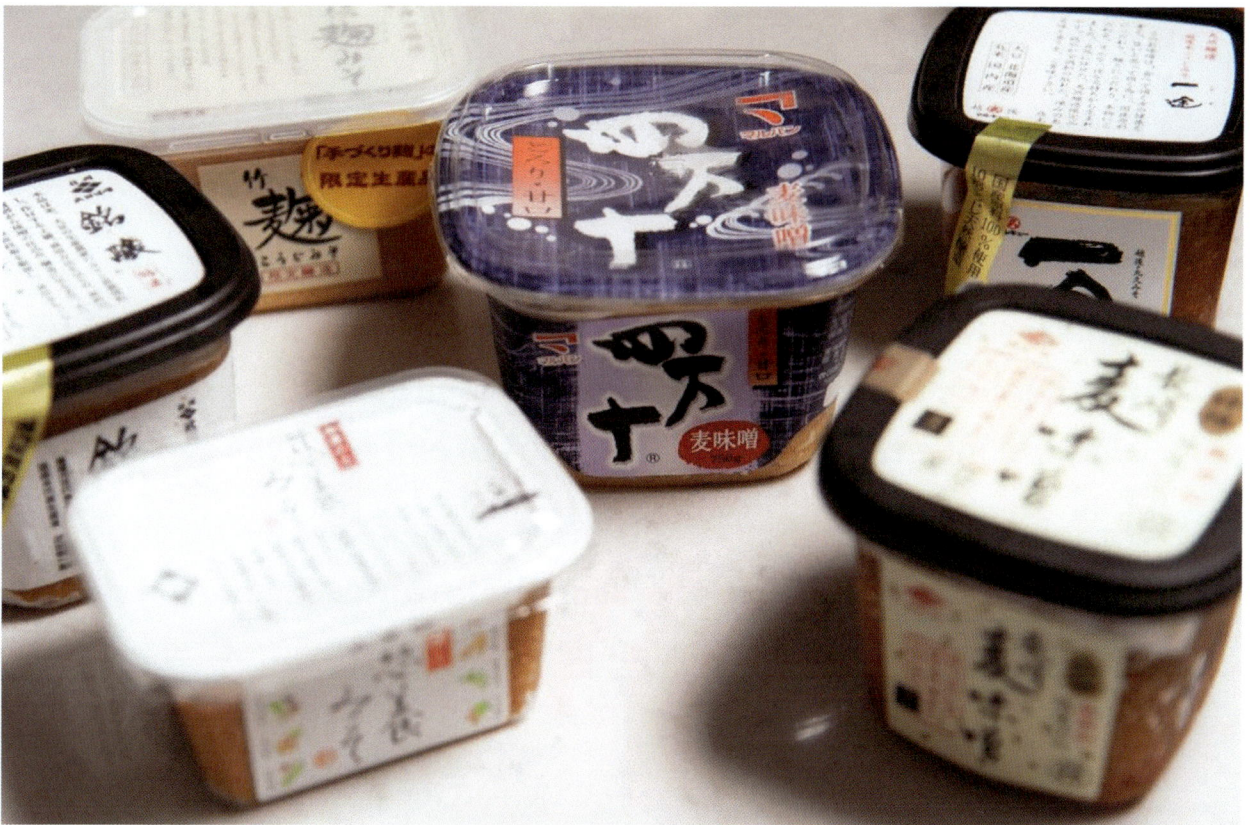

Different types of miso paste

Satou 砂糖 (white sugar)

You may have noticed salt isn't used that much in Japanese food. Most of the flavor either comes from the ingredients themselves, or from soy sauce, dashi or other seasonings. The use of sugar may surprise you, though it depends on what you're making. For example, many recipes for nimono (煮物 simmered foods) call for sugar because it helps to balance the salty, savory flavor.

Sometimes it's important to have a well-rounded flavor in terms of sweet and savory. In Japanese, this is called amakarai (甘辛い sweet and spicy/savory).

Okome お米 (rice)

A lot of Japanese rice is grown in America and exported to Japan. If you can find it, shinmai (新米 newly-harvested rice) tends to have better flavor and aroma.

Premium rice is well worth the additional few dollars per pound, in terms of flavor, texture and especially the aroma. Good quality rice can be enjoyed plain, without any seasoning. Try it yourself and see if you can appreciate the difference.

While there are many varieties of short grain (white and brown) rice, you'd be really hard pressed to tell a difference between them so I wouldn't worry much about this.

Genmai (玄米 brown rice) is what you'll need for the recipes in this book. As you may know brown rice is more nutritious than white rice with plenty of vitamins, minerals, protein, and fiber. It's also a whole food!

Other Japanese ingredients you may want to use

- Daizu (大豆 dried soy beans) for making soy milk, okara, and yuba
- Nerigoma (練り胡麻 sesame paste or tahini)
- Kudzuko (葛粉 arrowroot starch)
- Koyadoufu(高野豆腐 freeze dried tofu)
- Kanpyou (干瓢 dried bitter gourd)
- Umeboshi (梅干し pickled plum)
- Komekouji (米麹 aspergillus incoulated rice)
- Shiokouji (塩麹 salted fermented rice)
- Kanten (寒天 agar) powder or stick forms

Where to find Japanese ingredients

If you don't have a Japanese or Asian grocery store near you, all of these items can be ordered online. For links to important books on food, Amazon shopping lists, online Japanese grocery stores and additional Japanese cooking resources, visit **alldayieat.com/go/bookresources**.

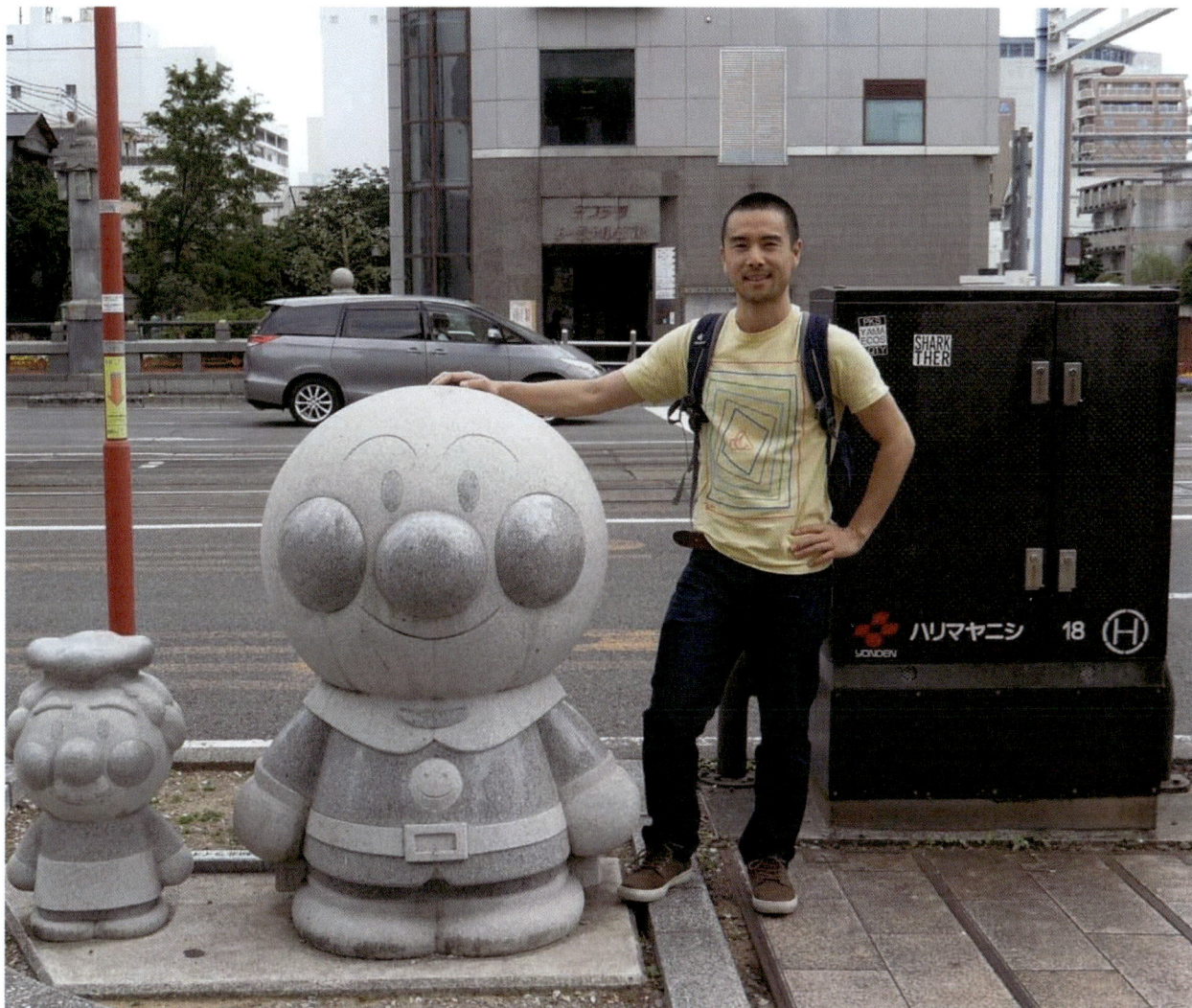

Anpanman and I, Kochi City, Japan

Shiitake konbu dashi
(Shiitake mushroom and kelp stock)
しいたけ昆布だし

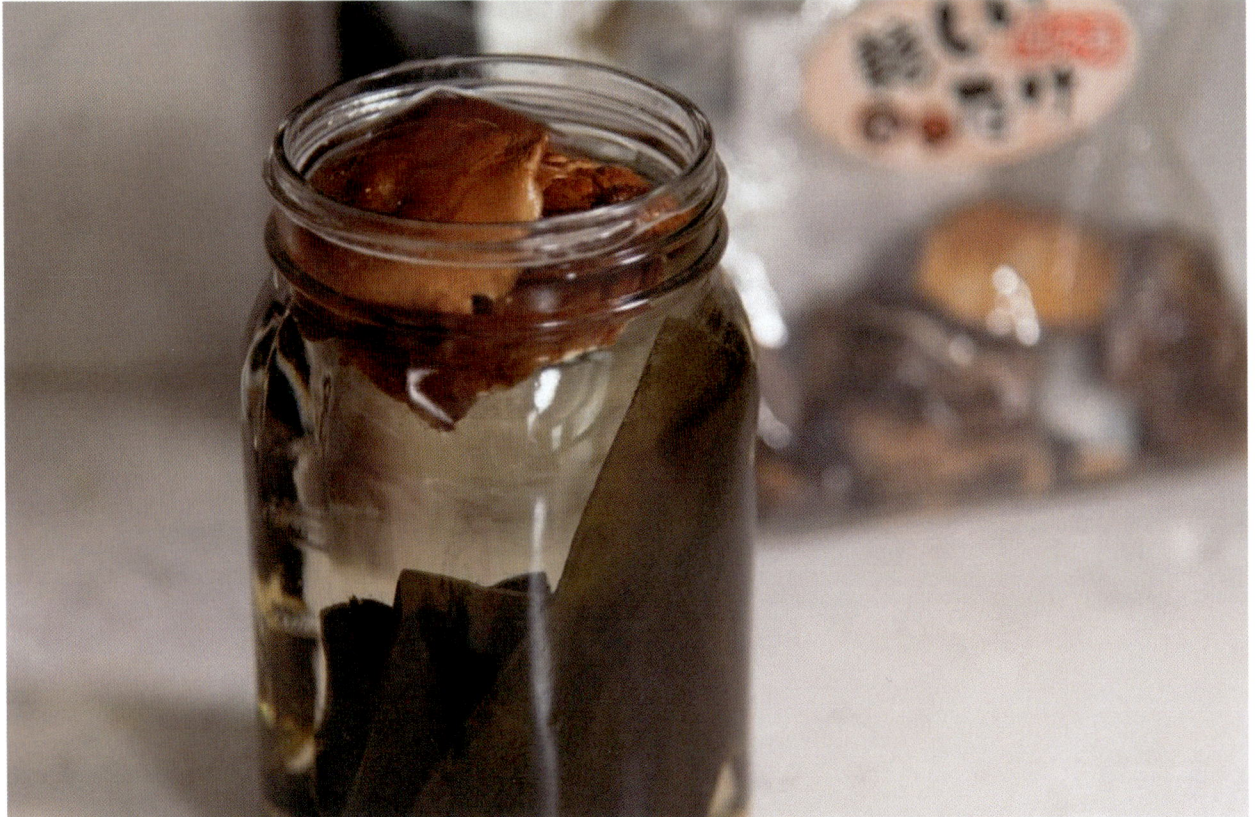

Dashi is one of the most important ingredients in Japanese cuisine. Like many other types of soup stock (e.g. vegetable, chicken or beef stock) dashi has many different uses. For plant-based dashi, you can use dried shiitake mushrooms alone or in combination with konbu (dried kelp). You can also use konbu by itself to make konbu dashi.

If you've never made dashi before, there are a two simple ways you can prepare it. One is the mizudashi method (cold water extraction) and the other is the nidashi method (hot water extraction). While hot water will generally result in a fuller and stronger flavored dashi, the mizudashi method is good enough, especially if you're not in a rush or prefer its convenience.

There are also many different types of konbu which have slightly different flavors and characteristics. The same thing goes with shiitake mushrooms. If you have the opportunity, try the different types and see if you can taste the difference. It's always fun to try new things, isn't it?

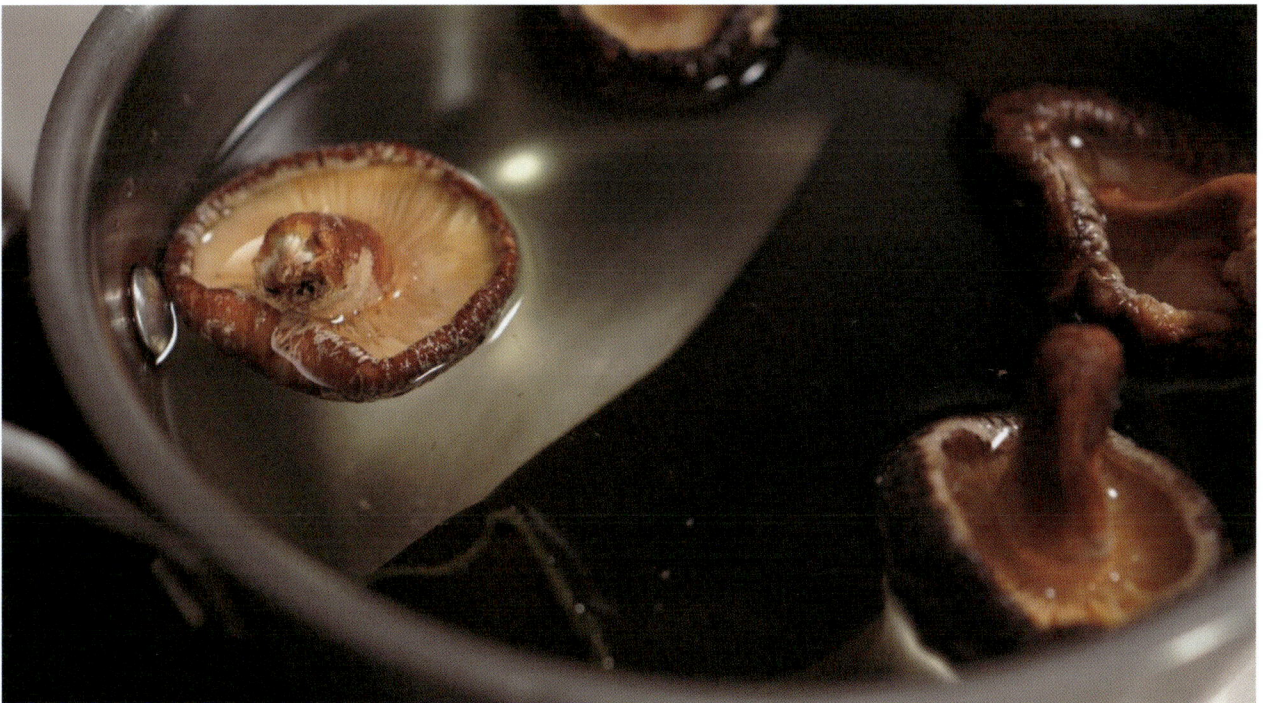

Rehydrated konbu and shiitake (before cooking)

Makes 4 cups

Ingredients

* 10g dried konbu (4 x 5 in. piece)
* 5 g dried shiitake mushrooms 3-6 pieces
* 4 cups water

Mizudashi (水だし cold water method)

1. Add the konbu, dried shiitake and water to an airtight container.
2. Allow to sit in the refrigerator overnight.
3. The next day, strain to remove the konbu and shiitake. Use immediately or store in the fridge and use or freeze within 2-3 days.

Nidashi (煮だし simmered method)

1. Add the konbu, shiitake, and water to a medium saucepan. Let it rest and rehydrate for at least 30 minutes.
2. Heat on medium heat and bring the stock to just before a boil. You'll notice tiny bubbles forming around the konbu. This indicates that you'll soon need to turn the heat down and maintain that state (avoiding a boil). Maintain the heat at this level for at least 10 minutes before removing the konbu from the pot.**
3. Continue cooking the shiitake mushrooms for another 20-30 minutes at a gentle simmer.
4. Strain and use immediately or store in the fridge and use or freeze within 2-3 days.

Tips:

* ****If you want to make konbu dashi**, the process is the same minus the shiitake. For the nidashi method you are finished making konbu dashi at step 2 after cooking the rehydrated konbu for 10 minutes!
* **If you want to make shiitake dashi**, the process is the same minus the konbu!
* Some people may lightly wipe dry konbu with a cloth to remove dirt or dust. This is optional and in my experience it doesn't affect the flavor, so I don't do it. Note that the white powder you see on the konbu is the good stuff (umami). You may lose some of it if you wipe too aggressively.

- Use a scale to weigh the dried konbu and dried shiitake. Both ingredients come in many different shapes and sizes and a scale helps you achieve a consistent flavor each time.
- Avoid breaking or cutting slits into your konbu prior to making dashi. Doing so can hasten release of bitter flavors and slime into your dashi.
- Avoid using high heat or cooking for longer than indicated. Overcooking/heating can cause bitter flavors and slime to be released into the broth.
- Whichever method you use, remember to save the konbu and shiitake. Both ingredients can be reused for something like tsukudani 佃煮 (soy sauce seasoned foods) or cut into small pieces and added to your miso soup or stew. Because it has been used for dashi, you can now refer to it as dashigara konbu (**だしがら昆布** dashi empty konbu) or dashigara shiitake(**だしがら椎茸** (dashi empty shiitake).
- For the mizudashi method specifically, there's a lot of flavor left in the ingredients because the mizudashi method is passive. This is something worth remembering when deciding how to repurpose your dashi ingredients in other dishes.

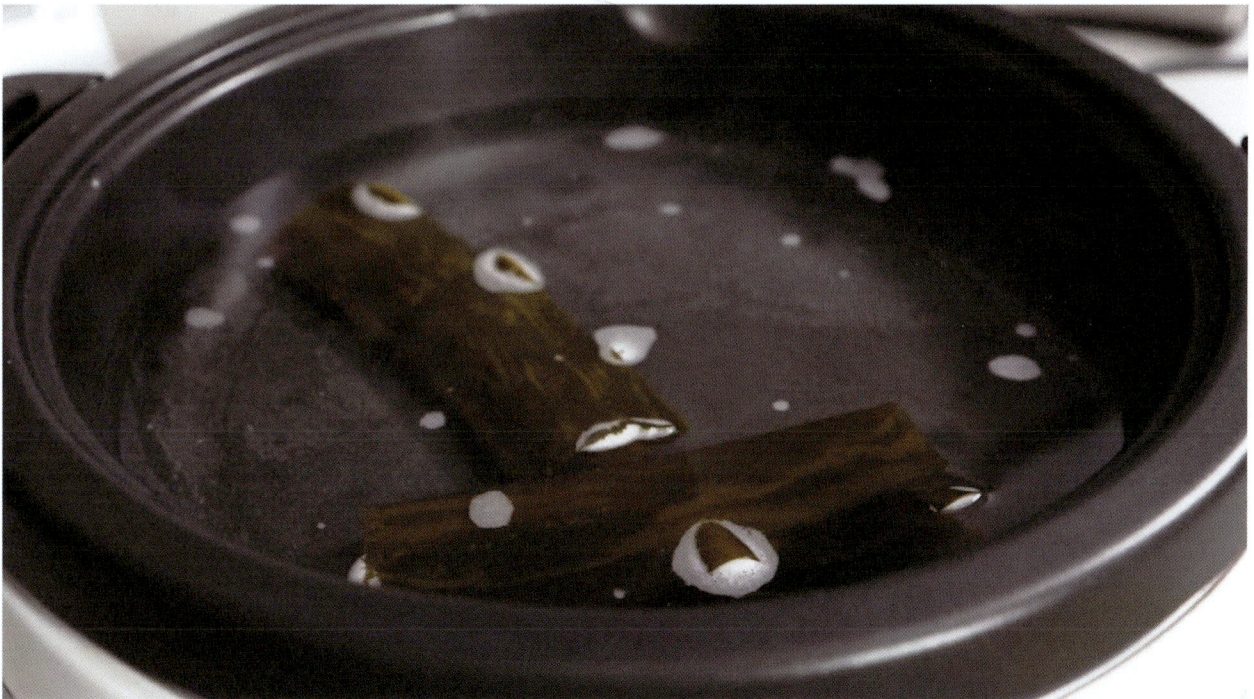

Rehydrating konbu

Okara misoshiru (Okara miso soup)
おから味噌汁

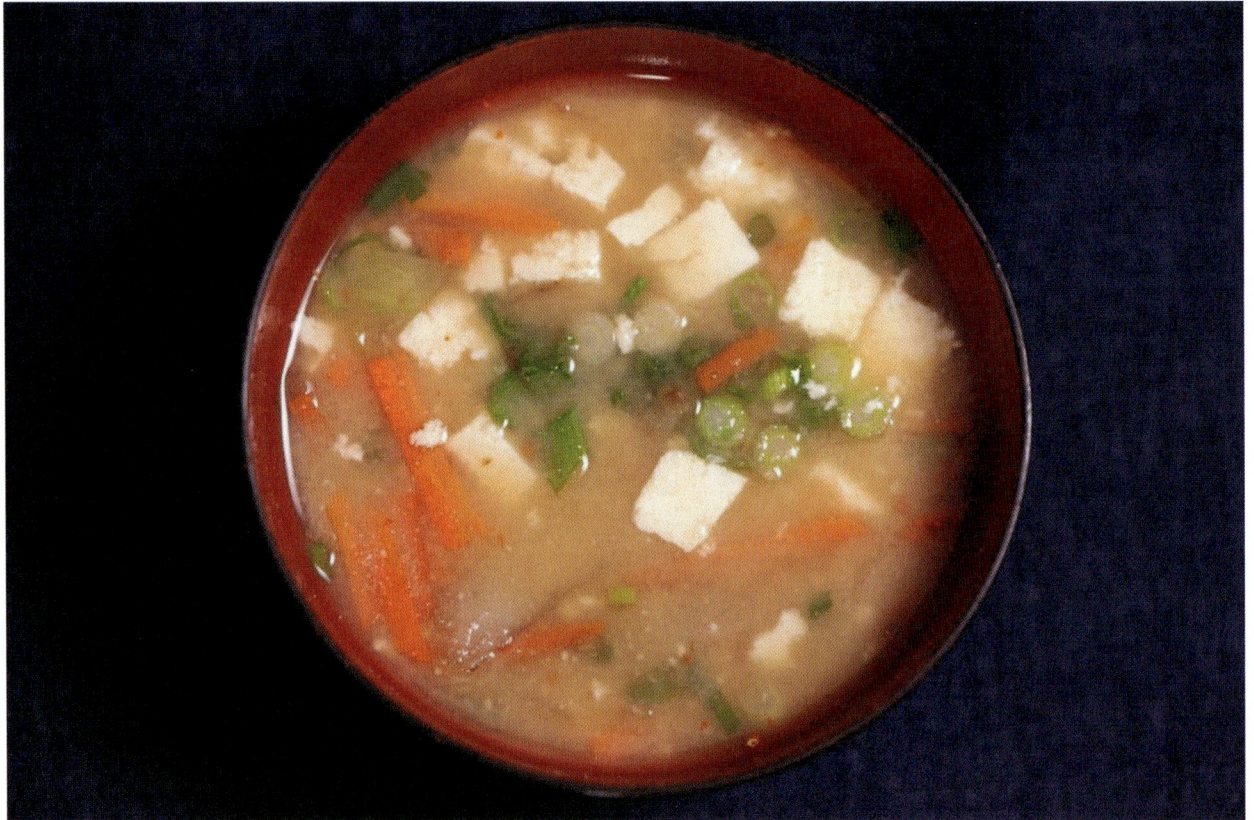

There's nothing quite like a good misoshiru (味噌汁 miso soup). And when you add something as nutritious and filling as okara (おから leftover soy bean pulp from making soy milk), it's just that much better!

Okara has many uses in both baking and cooking. And it's the perfect way to thicken up your miso soup while reusing the leftovers from your homemade soy milk. It has a very neutral flavor and will not only improve the texture, but also make your soup more nutritious and filling!

Makes 3-4 servings

Ingredients

- 2 cups dashi
- 1 cup carrots, cut into match sticks
- 1 cup gobo, (burdock root) sasagaki (small pointed strips)*
- 1 cup green onions, chopped
- ½ block tofu (7 oz.), drained and cut into small blocks
- ¼ cup okara, (leftover soy bean pulp from making soy milk)
- 2 Tbsps miso paste

Directions

1. Heat 2 cups dashi in a small saucepan and add in the carrots and gobo.
2. Cook for 2-3 minutes until slightly softened.
3. Next add in green onions and tofu, bring to a boil.
4. Add in okara and reduce heat to a simmer.
5. Once heated through, stir in and dissolve miso paste and serve immediately!

Tips:

- *For gobo, scrape off outside skin using back edge of knife to remove excess dirt; the skin has flavor and nutrients so you don't want to remove all of it.
- Sasagaki (ささがき) is a Japanese cutting technique where you cut a vegetable into small pointed strips using a knife. You can think of it like sharpening a pencil, shaving off one little bit at a time. Cut each piece into a bowl of water to remove bitter flavors and prevent oxidation (discoloring). Strain thoroughly before adding to pot. Visit alldayieat.com/go/bookresources for a mini video tutorial on this cutting technique.
- Always add in miso paste at the very end of cooking so that you protect the aroma. If you boil it and or leave the hot soup uncovered, you'll lose some of the aroma. After serving, if you have any left in the pot, make sure to cover it with a lid. If you don't have traditional Japanese bowls with lids, don't worry! Just wait to serve it until just before you're about to eat so you can enjoy the savory aroma of your miso soup.
- You can substitute other vegetables too if you'd like, for example, spinach, daikon radish, and wakame (わかめ dried seaweed).

- The okara adds a nice thickness to the soup, much thicker than your average miso soup. If you aren't keen on the texture, you could try using half the amount. And if you love it, consider adding another tablespoon or two!
- If you don't have okara, another way to get a similar consistency is to use an equal amount of cooked brown or yellow potato mashed with a fork. Though not as nutritious, it will help to thicken up the soup and provide a similar texture.

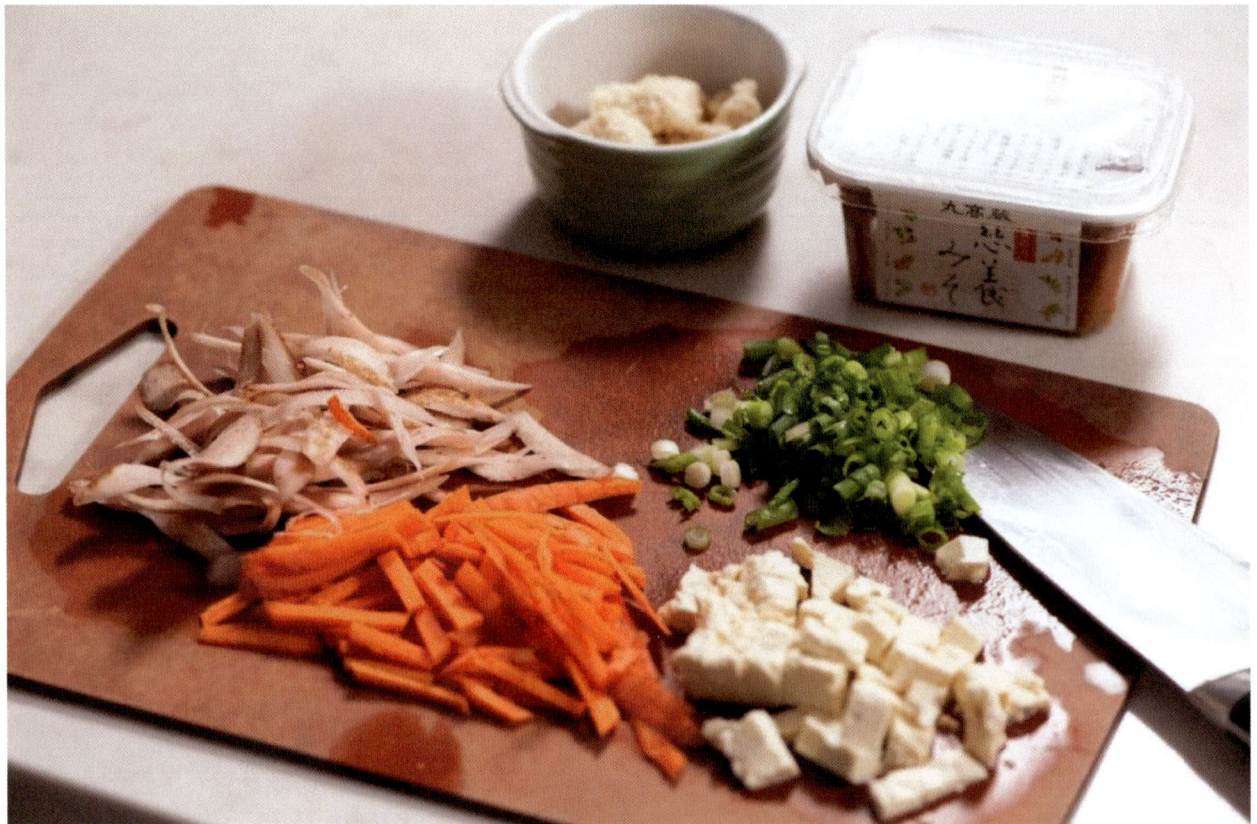

Ingredients for okara misoshiru

Kenchinjiru (Vegetable soup)
けんちん汁

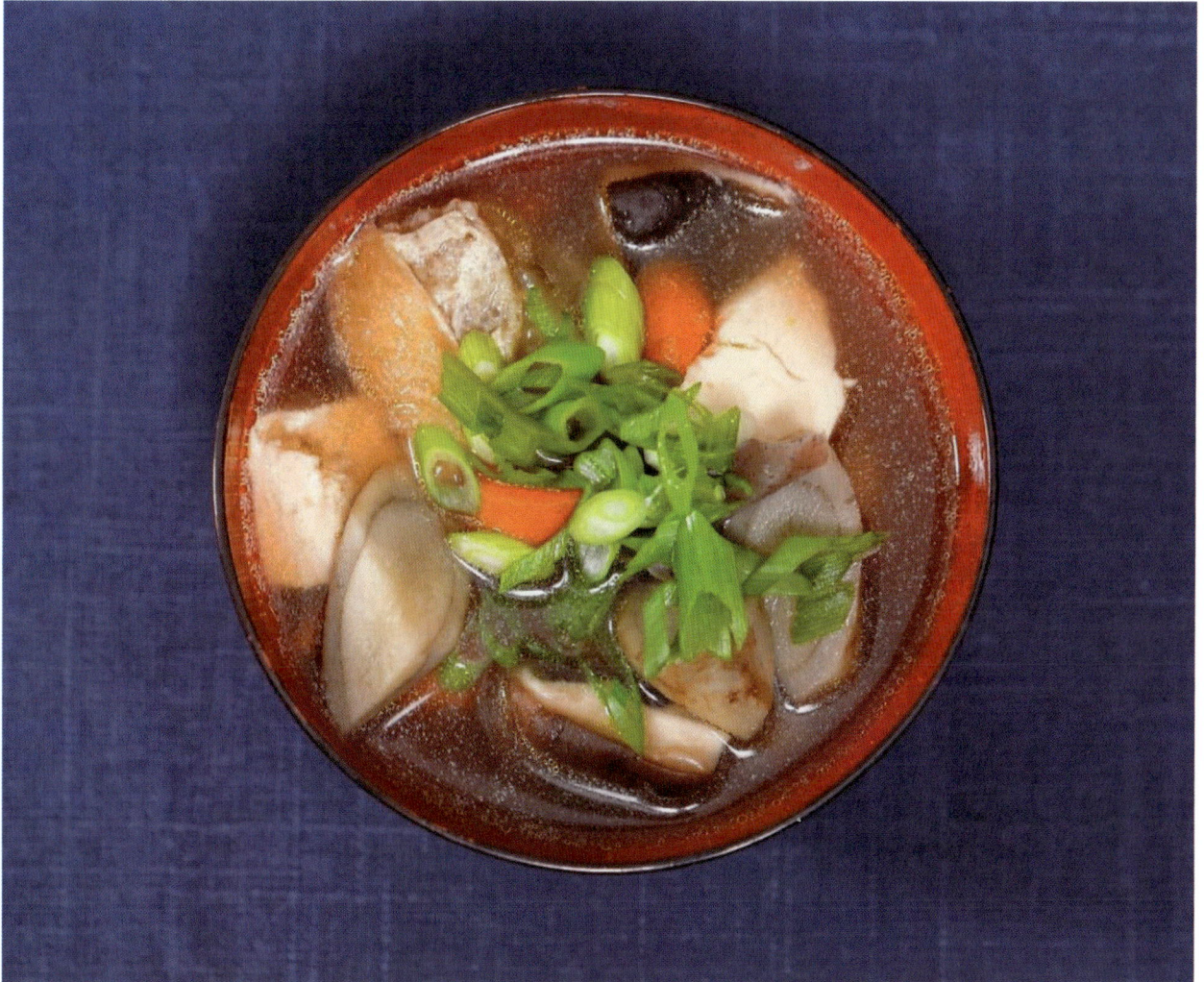

What makes a good vegetable soup better than others?

For me, it's when you can taste the vegetables for what they are. While there are times when you might not want to taste individual components, this is one occasion where you do.

And they're especially delicious in combination with each other too.

Makes 5-6 servings

Ingredients

- 4-5 in. piece of daikon radish, sliced into half moon pieces, ¼ in. thick
- 1 ½ cups gobo, (burdock root) rangiri*
- 1 tsp fresh ginger, sliced
- 1 cup carrots, rangiri**
- 1 Tbsp olive or sesame oil
- 1 cup fresh shiitake mushrooms, sliced
- 2 pieces aburaage, (fried tofu skins, 2 x 6 in. each) sliced
- ½ block konnyaku (3.5 oz), parboiled and torn with a spoon into small pieces
- ½ block tofu (7 oz.), drained and cut into bite size pieces
- 4 cups dashi
- 1 Tbsp mirin
- 2 Tbsps sake
- 1 ½ Tbsps soy sauce

Toppings- chopped green onions sesame seeds (toasted and crushed), black and/or white pepper, shichimi or sansho pepper

Directions

1. Using a large pot, add the oil and cook carrots, daikon, and gobo for 2-3 minutes.
2. Add in the ginger, shiitake, aburaage, konnyaku, tofu, dashi, mirin, and sake. Cover partially with a lid and simmer for about 10 minutes.
3. Add the soy sauce and simmer for another 5 minutes partially covered.
4. Serve with desired toppings as a side or with a bowl of rice for a complete meal!

Tips:

- *For gobo, scrape off outside skin using back edge of knife to remove excess dirt. If not using immediately, soak cut pieces in a bowl of water to remove bitter flavors and prevent oxidation.

- **Rangiri (乱切り random cut), is a cutting technique where you rotate a round vegetable ¼ inch at a time and then cut it at an angle. This helps to increase the surface area for better flavor and even cooking. Visit alldayieat.com/go/bookresources for a mini video tutorial on this cutting technique.

- Parboiling the konnyaku for 2-3 minutes helps to remove some of the unpleasant flavor and smell along with some of the water inside. Tearing the konnyaku either by hand or with a spoon helps to increase the surface area to allow for the broth flavor to be absorbed better.

- For the aburaage, you can reduce some of the oil you eat by parboiling it for 1-2 minutes in water and then draining before using. The trade off is you'll lose a little bit of flavor from the oil. If you do this, make sure to squeeze out all the water it absorbed before adding it to the soup.

- When cooking the konsai (根菜 root vegetables such as daikon radish, carrot and gobo), consider allowing them to brown slightly for extra flavor and umami.

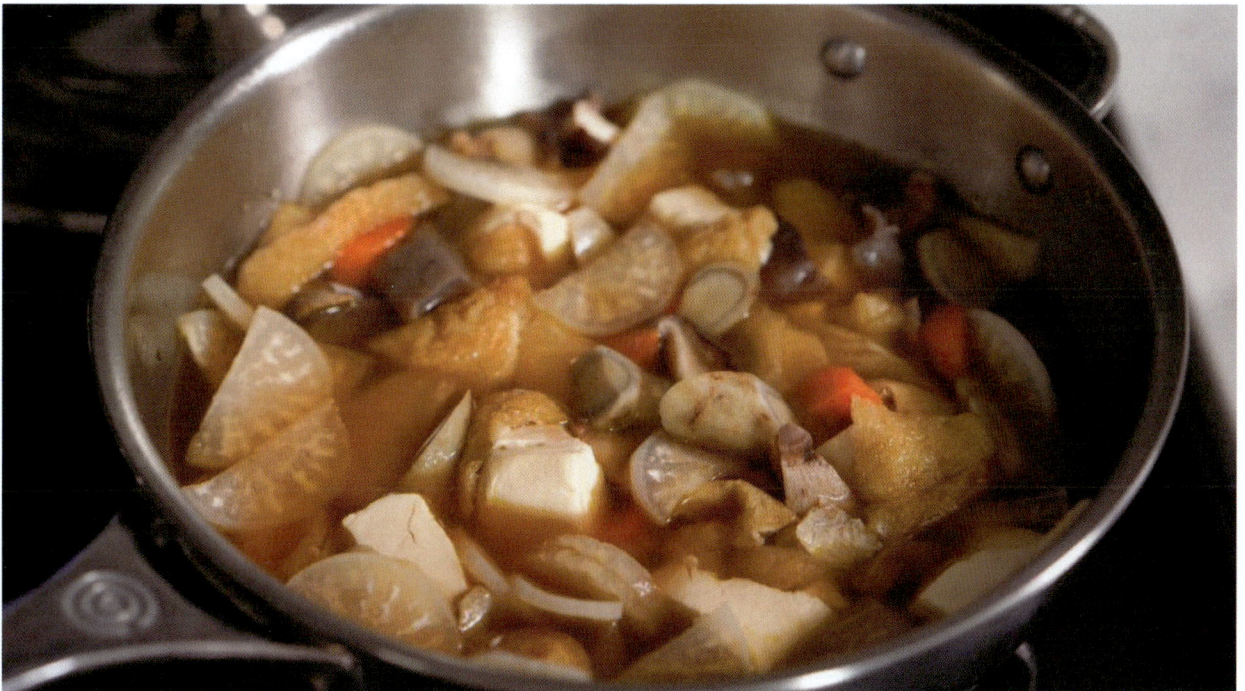

Simmering the kenchinjiru

Kurogomadoufu (Black sesame tofu)

黒ゴマ豆腐

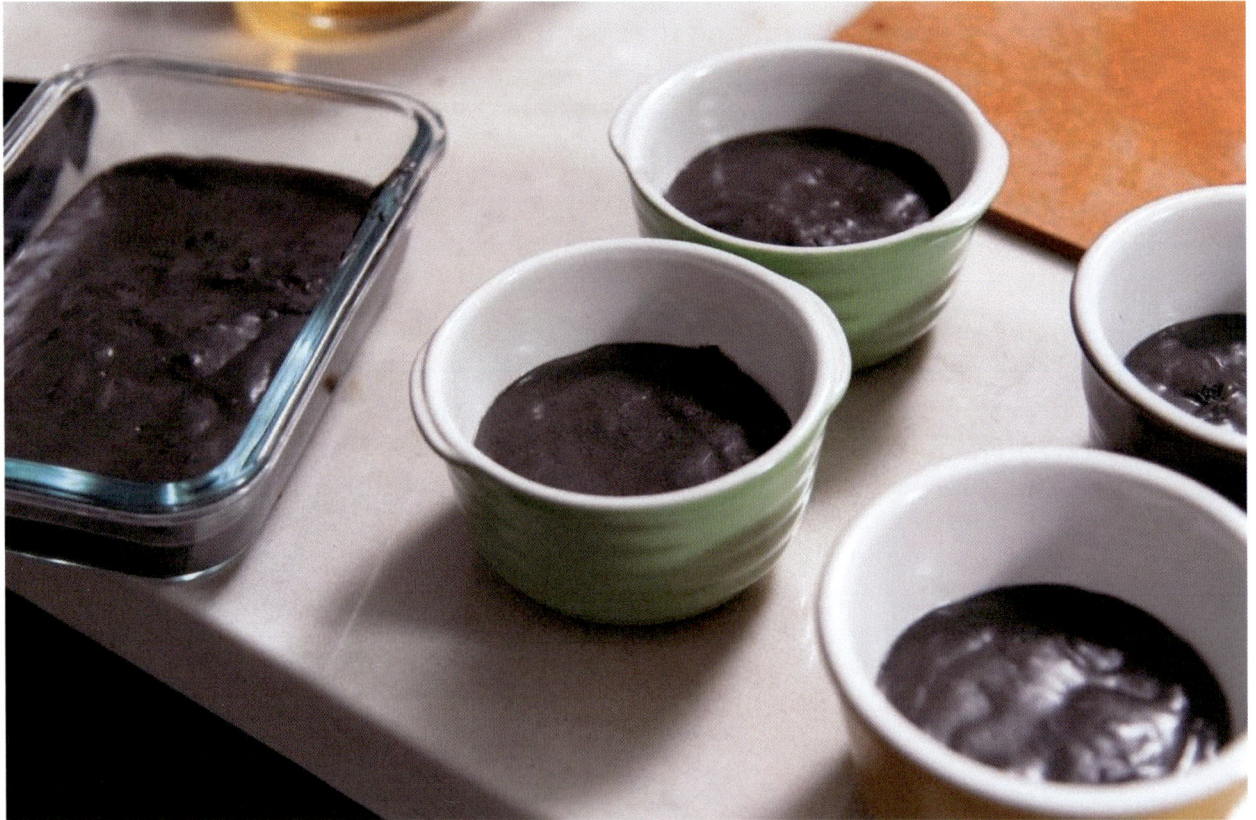

When you hear 'tofu', chances are the first thing that comes to mind is tofu made from soy beans.

Well, you might be surprised to learn there are many different types of 'tofu' made from non-soy bean ingredients. And this particular 'tofu' is made from sesame seeds!

Gomadoufu (胡麻豆腐 sesame tofu) is one of my favorite side dishes for a Japanese meal.

This is an extremely simple and delicious dish that is creamy and full of flavor, and absolutely sure to impress those who enjoy sesame.

Just add a few fresh ingredients like grated ginger, green onions or wasabi for a very satisfying experience.

You can use white or black sesame paste for different flavors. And if you're up to it, you can even make the paste from scratch, but it is a lot of work!

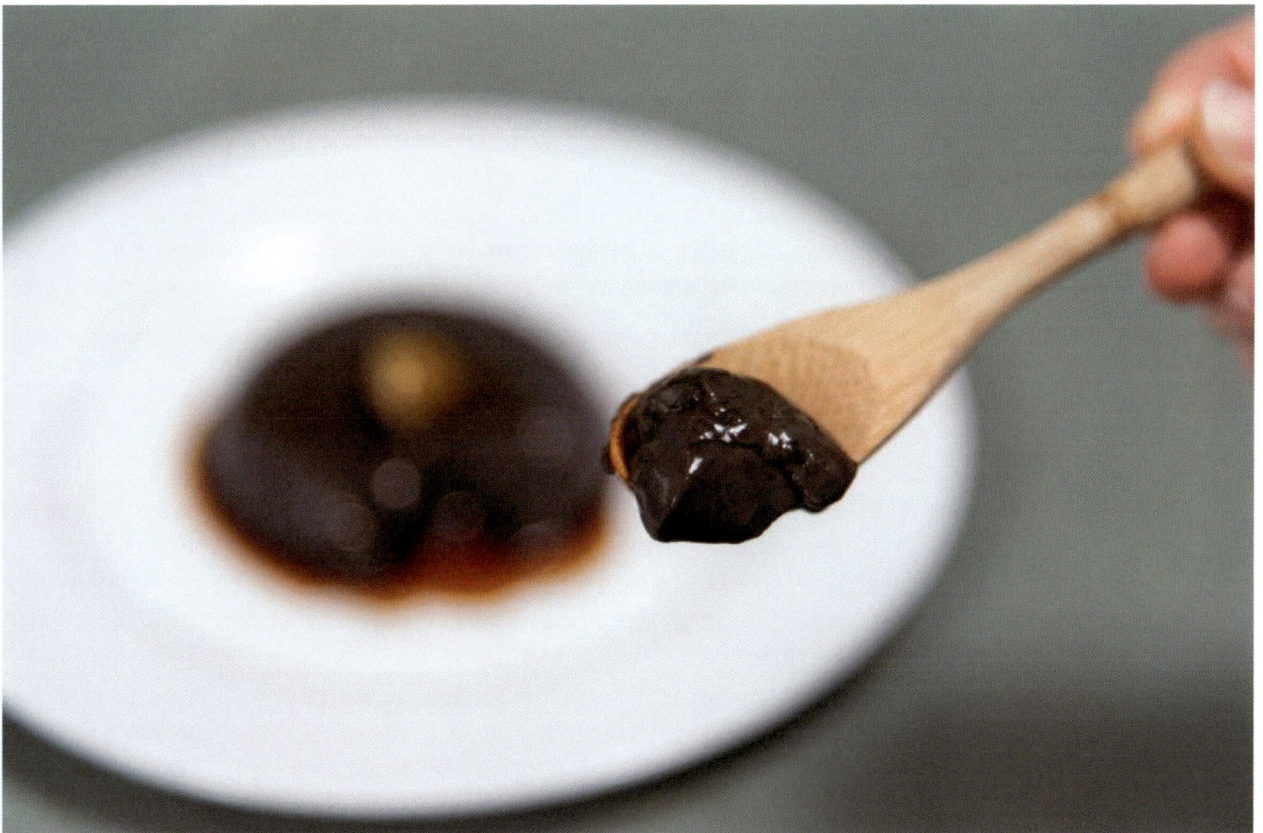

Kurogomadoufu with wasabi and soy sauce

Makes 6 servings

Ingredients

- 2 ½ cups konbu dashi, at room temperature
- 2-3 Tbsps black nerigoma, black sesame paste (60 g)
- 3-4 Tbsps kudzuko, arrowroot starch (50 g); alternatively potato starch

Toppings - wasabi, freshly grated ginger, soy sauce, chopped green onion

Directions

1. Combine kudzuko with 2/3 of the dashi using an immersion or regular blender.
2. Once there are no clumps, add all the sesame paste and blend again.
3. Add the remaining dashi and blend once more and transfer to a small saucepan.
4. Cook the mixture on medium low heat, for 12-15 minutes **stirring constantly to prevent any clumping.**
5. Transfer the mixture to ramekins, or a large heatproof container.
6. Allow to cool and then chill in the refrigerator to set, at least 2 hours.
7. Top with desired toppings and enjoy!

Tips:

- Tahini can be used in place of black or white nerigoma.
- To be consistent with the texture, weigh the sesame paste and the starch (especially if the kudzuko is in the form of small pieces rather than powder).
- If you're using freshly made (hot) konbu dashi, allow it to cool to room temperature before using. Otherwise, the heat may begin to activate the starch and cause the mixture to thicken too quickly.
- As the mixture begins to thicken, if you don't stir constantly, you'll end up with clumps. You may be able to smooth out the mixture with an immersion blender, but might be more difficult if you're using a regular blender... so tend to it closely!
- If you want a softer gomadoufu, use a little less (1-2 teaspoons less) kudzuko.
- If you want a richer gomadoufu, use a little more (2-3 teaspoons additional) nerigoma.
- Gomadoufu is meant to be eaten as a small dish alongside other small dishes. For example, if you stay at a temple in Japan you might get this as part of your Shojin Ryouri(精進料理 Buddhist cuisine) meal. You'd be served this along side miso soup, a bowl of rice, a small piece of tofu, simmered seasonal vegetables, or some pickles.
- Gomadoufu will keep for a few days. If you prefer, it can be eaten cool, at room temperature or slightly warm (microwaved for 20 seconds for a softer texture).

Kabocha nimono
(Simmered kabocha squash)
南瓜煮物

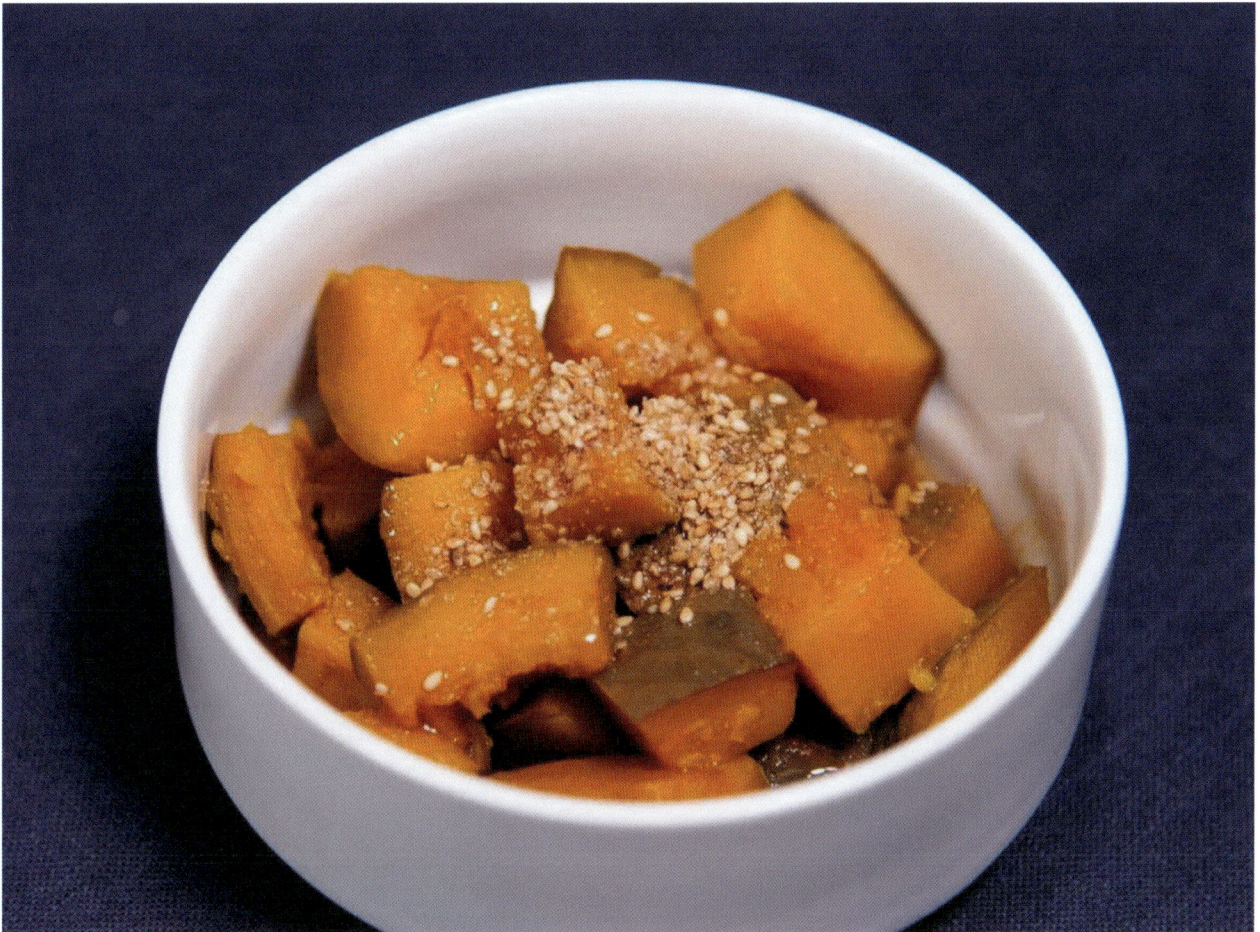

Nimono (煮物) means 'simmered thing' in Japanese. And while most vegetables can be simmered, the inherent sweetness and creaminess naturally found in kabocha makes for one of the best simmered dishes you may ever make. It's delicious when served warm and also served cold   as part of your obento (お弁当 box lunch). This kabocha nimono might be your new favorite way to enjoy kabocha. It's definitely one of mine!

Makes 4-6 servings

Ingredients

- ½ small kabocha, (~3 cups of cut pieces)
- 1 cup konbu dashi
- 1-2 tsps kokutou, Okinawan black sugar; alternatively muscovado or brown sugar
- 1 Tbsp sake
- 1 Tbsp soy sauce

Toppings – toasted and ground sesame seeds and or sesame oil

Directions

1. Soften the kabocha by microwaving it on high for 4-5 minutes.
2. Once it has cooled, cut it open and remove top and bottom stems, seeds, and pith. Cut it into bite size pieces.
3. Using a medium sauce pan, add the kabocha, dashi, sugar, sake, and soy sauce and bring to a gentle simmer.
4. Cover with an otoshibuta (or leave partially covered if not using) and cook for 15-20 minutes, or until liquid has reduced by half. If desired, continue cooking for a more concentrated broth.
5. Use a chopstick to test for doneness. (If you can easily pierce through, it's done.)
6. Serve 2-4 pieces per person, top with sesame seeds or oil if desired.

Tips:

- You can reduce the broth all the way for a more concentrated flavor, but I prefer to have a little leftover. Just a few spoonfuls of broth is all you'd need for each serving.
- Shave a layer of skin off each piece which helps to infuse each kabocha piece with flavor and makes for a unique presentation style. Visit alldayieat.com/go/bookresources for a video tutorial on how to accomplish this.
- For the ultimate flavor in each bite, allow the kabocha to cool down once so that the flavors are fully absorbed or wait until the next day if you're patient. This is a technique which applies not only to nimono, but also Japanese curry too... Gaman dekiru? (**我慢できる?** Can you wait?)

Using an otoshibuta (落し蓋 drop lid) for nimono

- While an otoshibuta is not required, it's often used for simmered dishes like this one.
- There are several reasons why you might want to consider using one. An otoshibuta is designed to circulate the aroma and flavor from the surface of the broth to the top of the otoshibuta and back down onto the food you're cooking. Essentially, it creates an aroma and flavor-packed 'rain' that comes down from the surface of the otoshibuta and onto the food you're simmering. Soaking and infusing it during the cooking process.
- I recommend you try this technique to compare the difference in flavor when using an otoshibuta and when not using one for simmered dishes.
- As you may know - you can make an otoshibuta from parchment paper-
  - Start with a large square piece (larger than your pot) and cut a round shape a slightly smaller than the diameter of your pot (so it fits inside) and then fold it in half.
  - Cut 4-5 long slits evenly spaced across the surface. Once you're ready to be simmer your food, unfold and place on top of the food. Visit alldayieat.com/go/bookresources for a mini video tutorial on how to make an otoshibuta from parchment paper!

Achieving a clear broth in nimono

- As you may know, presentation is an extremely important aspect of Japanese cuisine. If you're particular about the broth and want to keep it clear there are several things you can do:
  - Carve the edges of the kabocha pieces. This cutting technique is called mentori (**面取り** to bevel) and will prevent the kabocha from breaking off/dissolving and making the broth cloudy. This technique can be used for other vegetables like daikon radish and carrots in simmered dishes. Visit alldayieat.com/go/bookresources for a mini video tutorial on this cutting technique.
  - Align the kabocha pieces skin side down and use an appropriate size pot so that there isn't too much space in between the pieces so they stay in place.
  - Make sure not to boil the pieces because boiling will cause them to bump around and naturally disintegrate into the broth as they soften from cooking.

Koyadoufu nimono
(Simmered freeze dried tofu)
高野豆腐煮物

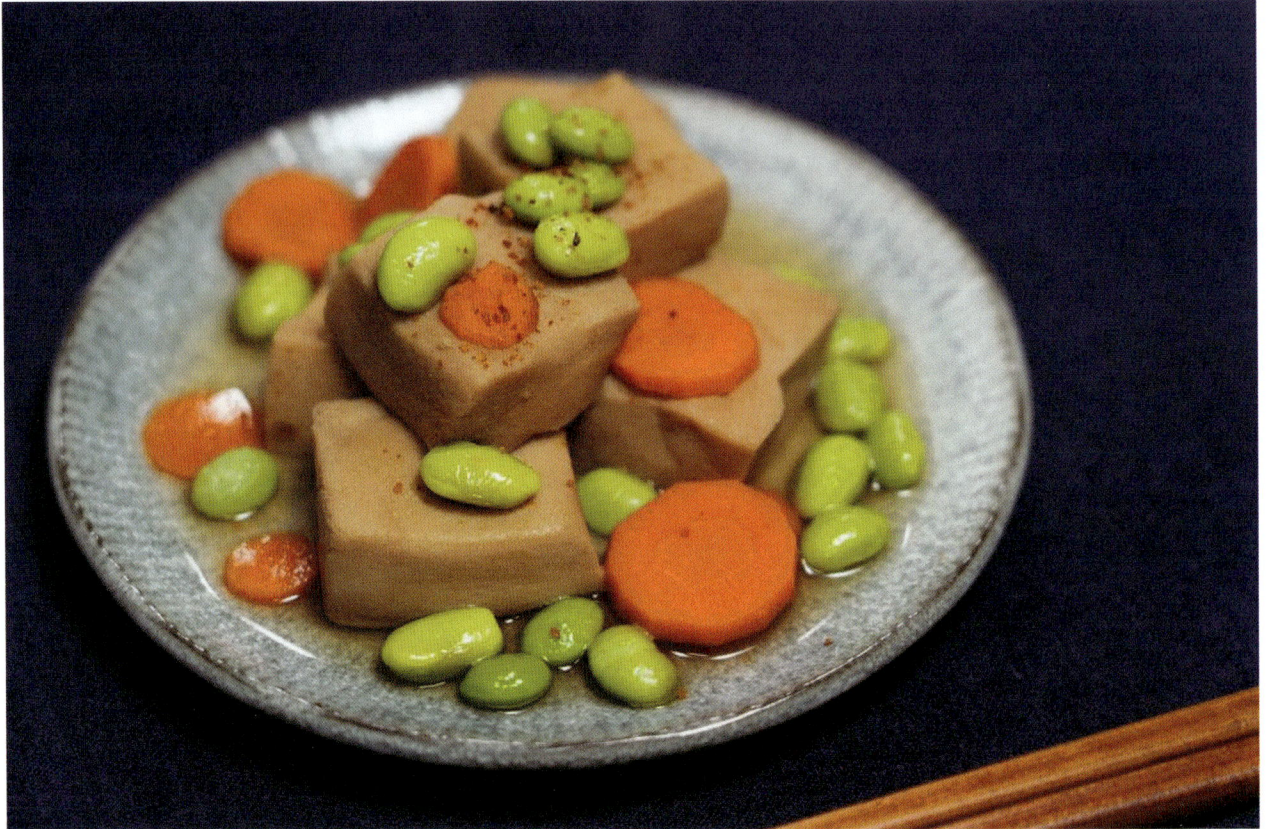

Mount Koya is a sacred mountain in Japan a short train ride away from the bustling city of Osaka. It's a small and quiet town and that's where this type of tofu originated from.

If you ever get a chance to visit, you can stay at one of many temples to enjoy Shojin Ryouri (精進料理 Buddhist cuisine). Some of the best plant-based food Japan has to offer!

Being freeze dried, koyadoufu offers a unique sponge-like consistency that soaks up any liquid seasoning.

Simmering it in a dashi-based broth is one of the most classic ways you can enjoy koyadoufu.

As you bite into each piece, you'll experience a burst of savory dashi flavor that floods your taste buds with happiness.

It's efficiency in accomplishing this is unlike any other food I've come across.

And as you can imagine, it would make for a very memorable and delicious experience for someone who's never had it before.

Just add a few green beans and carrots for color!

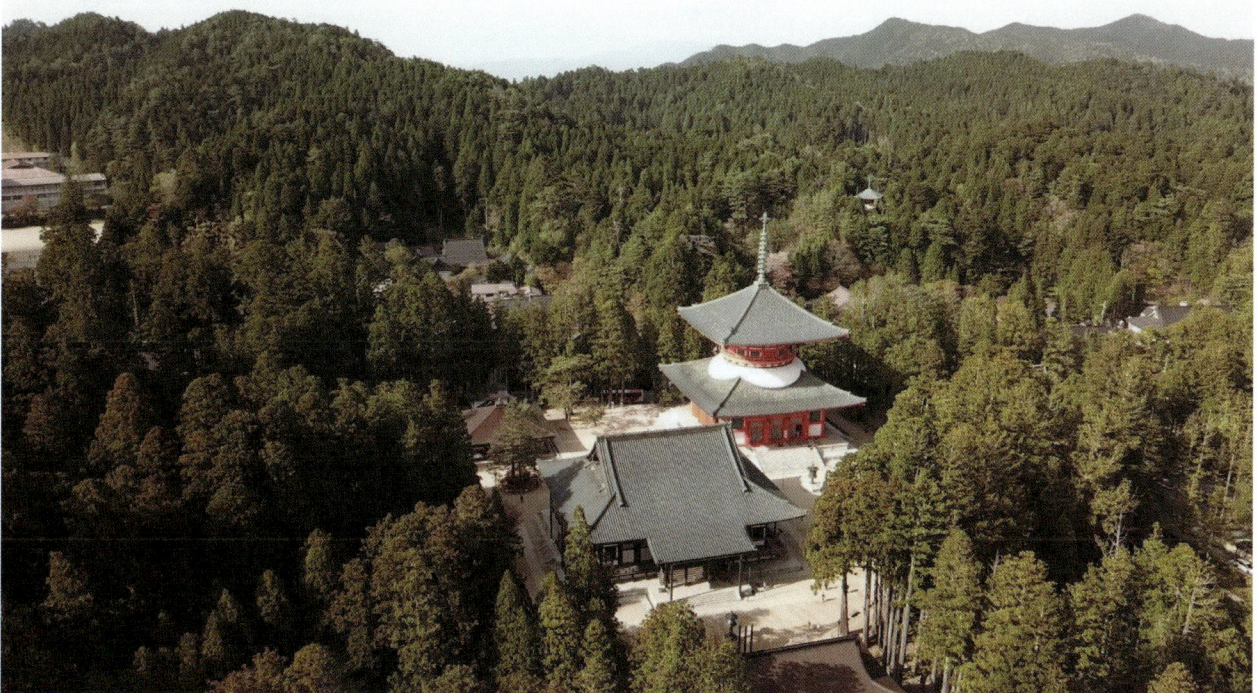

Konpon daito temple from above, Mount Koya, Japan

Makes 4–6 servings

Ingredients

- 6-8 squares koyadoufu, freeze dried tofu
- 1-2 carrots, sliced ¼ in. thick
- 1 cup edamame, shelled; alternatively, sugar snap peas, snow peas, or green beans
- 2 ½ cups dashi
- 2 Tbsps soy sauce
- 3 Tbsps mirin
- 3 Tbsps sake
- 2-3 Tbsps sugar
- Optional: 3-4 pieces dashigara shiitake (leftover shiitake from making dashi)

  Toppings– ichimi or shichimi red pepper, lemon zest

Directions

1. Rehydrate the koyadoufu blocks in warm water for about 10 minutes. Flip halfway to allow the other side to rehydrate if needed.
2. Squeeze out excess water into a bowl and cut into bite-size blocks.
3. Dip the dry blocks back into the same bowl with the soaking water (it's full of umami) to be reabsorbed.
4. Using a medium saucepan, combine the dashi, soy sauce, mirin, sake and sugar and bring to a boil.
5. Once boiling, add in the carrots, edamame, and koyadoufu blocks. Reduce heat to a simmer and cover with an otoshibuta or partially cover with a lid.
6. Cook for at least 15 minutes, or until liquid has reduced to your desired concentration. *If the liquid doesn't cover the ingredients, rotate at least halfway through to ensure even seasoning.*
7. Once the liquid has reduced, transfer to a small plate to serve and add desired toppings.

Tips:

- If you don't have koyadoufu on hand, you could use regular tofu that has been drained. If you do this, note that you may be missing the delicious burst of flavor you'd get from biting into the simmered koyadoufu. As you may know, regular tofu isn't that good of a vehicle for soaking up dashi broth.
- Koyadoufu can be used as a replacement for regular tofu in other dishes like miso soup. Just follow the first three steps to rehydrate it and use as desired.
- Do you like to play with your food or try different things? If so, here's a good opportunity for you! Consider playing with different colors, flavors and presentations:
  - For brown colors, you could also consider using different types of Japanese mushrooms such as shimeji, shiitake, enoki, or maitake. Other shades of brown could come from renkon (lotus root), gobo (burdock root) or konnyaku
  - For the greens, any green vegetable could work but I prefer to stick with green beans or peas for simple presentation.
  - For orange, consider cutting the carrot in different shapes like rangiri or in small match sticks. Kabocha also works well in this dish.
  - Like other nimono, you may find this dish tastes a little better the next day once the flavors have been fully absorbed by the ingredients.

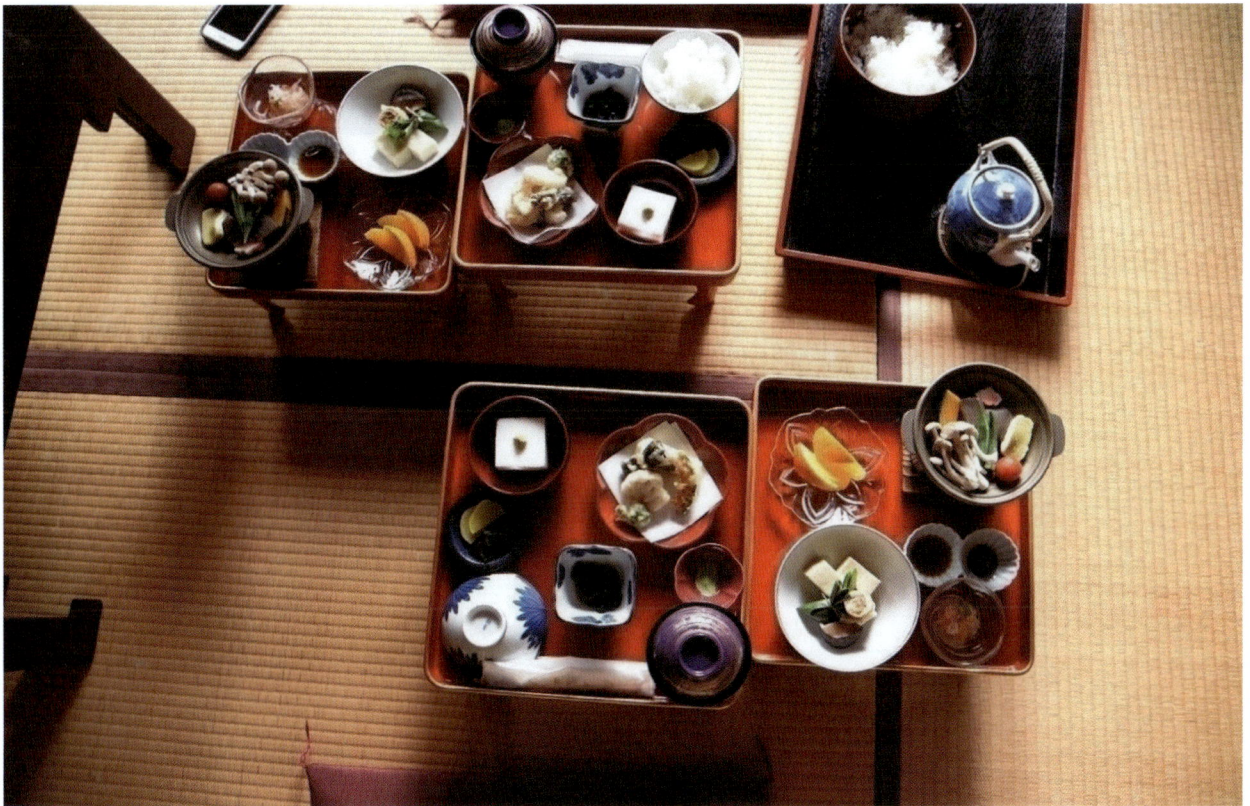

Shojin Ryouri dinner, Mount Koya, Japan

Daikon nimono (Simmered daikon radish)
大根煮物

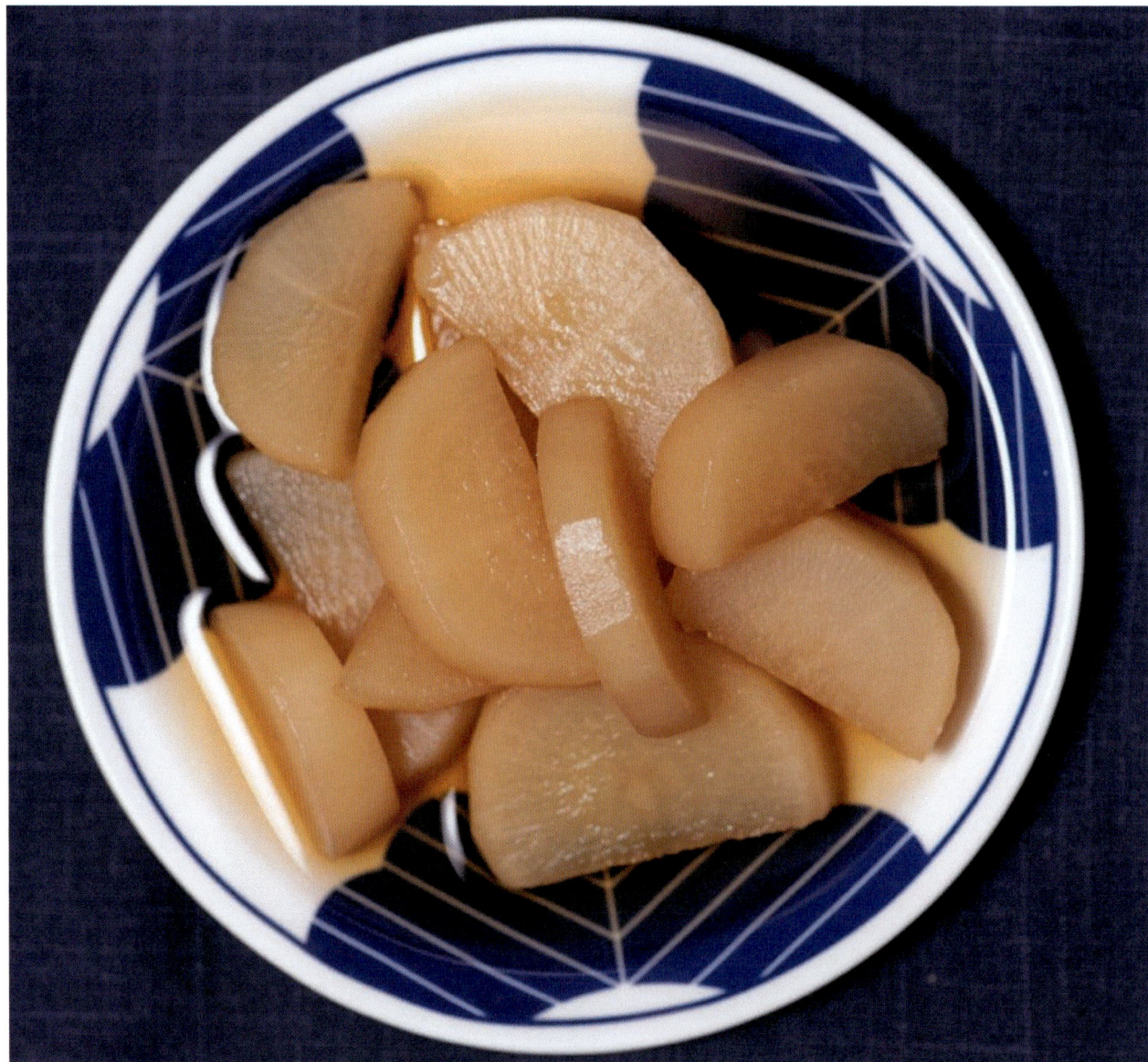

Daikon radish is another extremely versatile Japanese vegetable. While I thoroughly enjoy eating it as daikon oroshi (大根おろし freshly grated daikon), my second favorite way is to eat it simmered in a broth.

Whether the broth is seasoned with soy sauce or with just plain konbu dashi (like the furofuki daikon recipe on page 55), the way that it almost melts in your mouth, might make you completely change your perspective on the humble daikon radish! Especially if you take a few steps to pre-cook it using togijiru (とぎ汁 rice rinse water) or a little bit of sugar.

Togijiru or a sugared water both help to reduce the bitter flavors naturally found in daikon radish. Togijiru also helps to protect the white color of the daikon radish which can be important for the presentation of certain dishes.

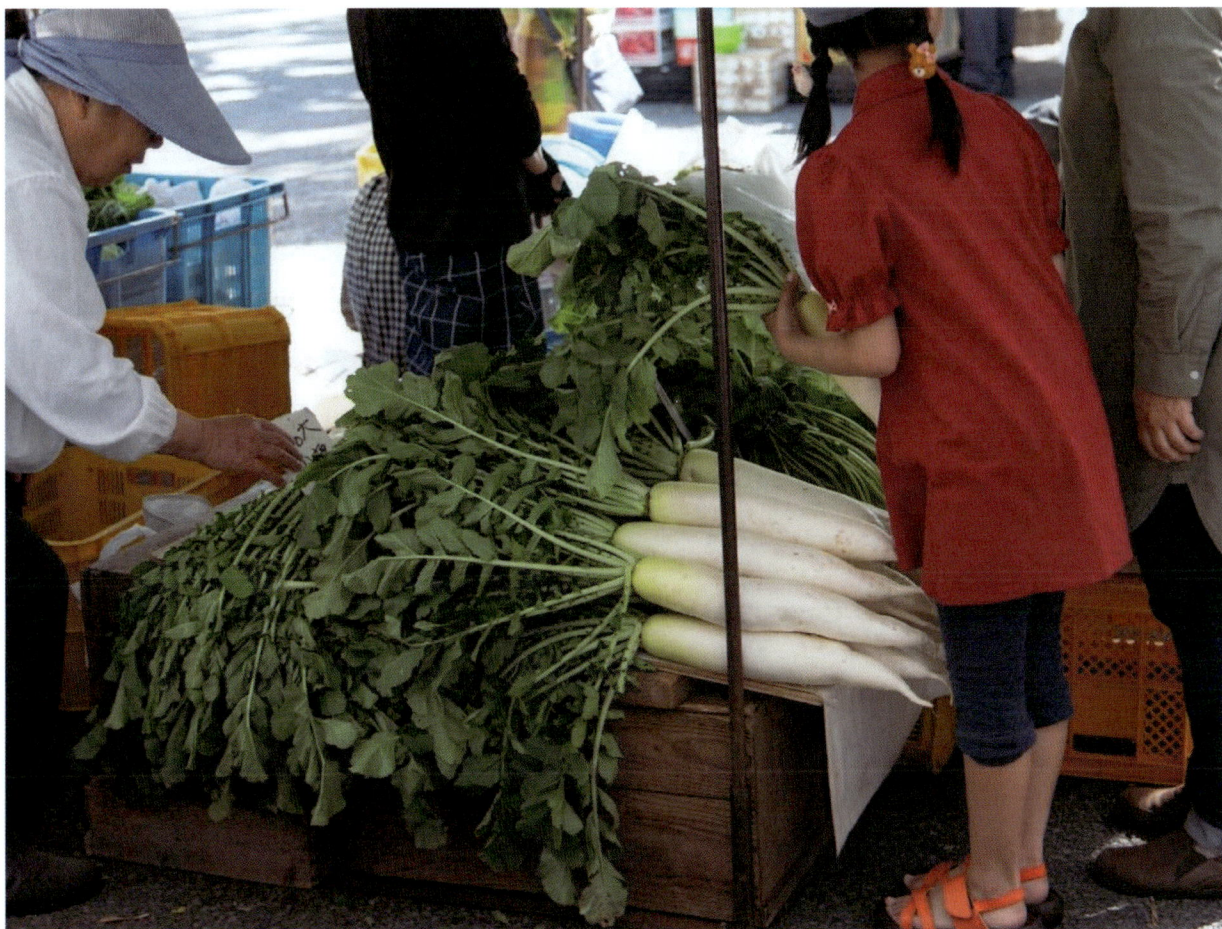

Large daikon radishes at the Sunday Market, Kochi City, Japan

Makes 6-8 servings

Ingredients

- 10-12 in. piece of daikon radish, peeled and cut into ½ in. thick rounds and then half-circles; mentori* optional
- 4 cups togijiru, cloudy white water from rinsing 2 cups of white rice
- 2 ½ cups konbu dashi
- 1 Tbsp sake
- 1 Tbsp mirin
- 2 Tbsps soy sauce

Toppings— ichimi or shichimi red pepper, lemon zest

Directions

1. Using a medium pot, add the togijiru and daikon pieces and bring to a boil.
2. Simmer for 20-30 minutes until you can pierce the daikon easily with a chopstick.
3. Strain the daikon, discarding the togijiru and return the daikon to the pot.
4. Add the konbu dashi, sake, and mirin. Bring to a gentle simmer and cover with an otoshibuta or partially cover with a lid. Cook for 15-20 minutes until liquid has reduced by about half.
5. Add the soy sauce and continue simmering for another 10-20 minutes with the otoshibuta or partially covered with a lid.
6. Taste the broth and if it's concentrated enough for you, it's done.
7. Serve warm with desired toppings and enjoy!

Tips:

- If you don't have togijiru on hand, use 1 tablespoon of sugar in 4 cups of water and cook the radish pieces until you can easily pierce them with a chopstick. This is an equally effective alternative to reduce the bitter flavors naturally found in daikon radish.
- Ensure you cut the daikon pieces as uniformly as possible for even cooking.
- For a clearer broth, use the techniques detailed in the kabocha nimono recipe tips on page 45:
  - use the mentori carving technique
  - align the foods in a way that minimizes movement .
  - avoid boiling the broth.
- As with other nimono (simmered dishes), consider using an otoshibuta to maximize the flavor and allow to cool down before eating so that the flavors are fully absorbed.

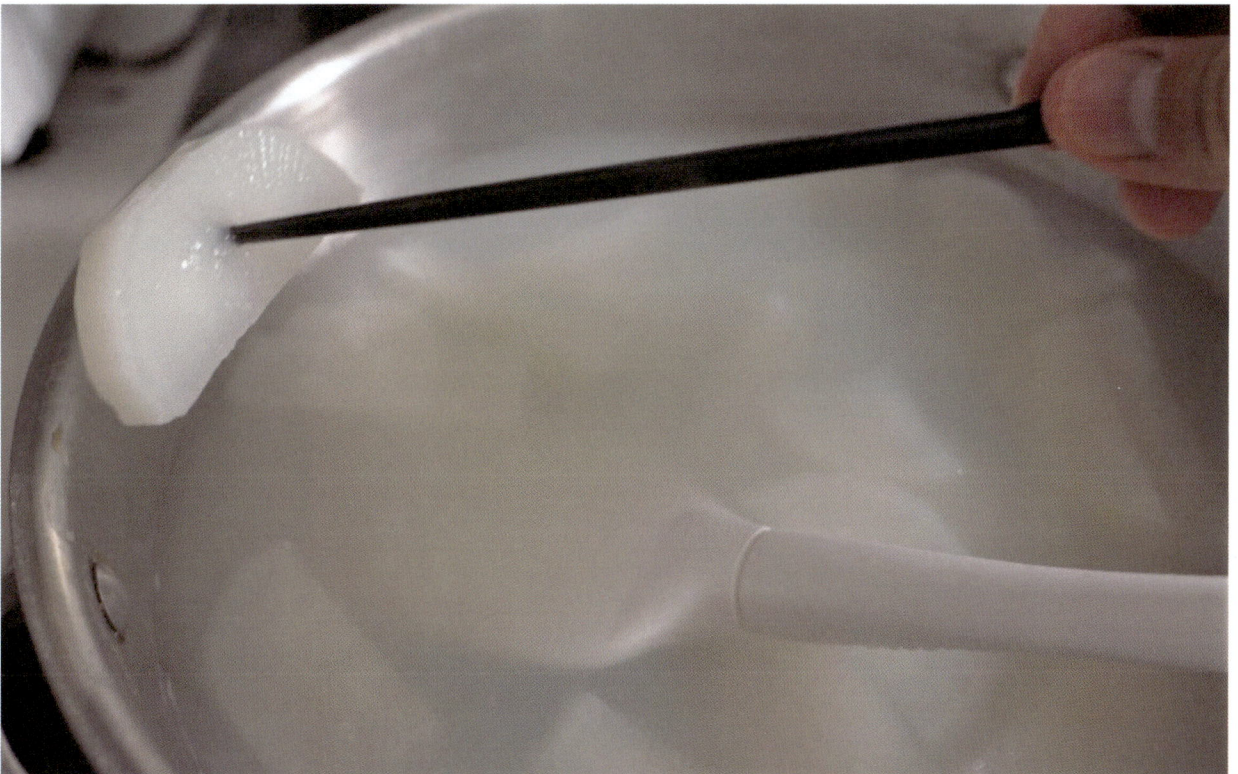

The chopstick test

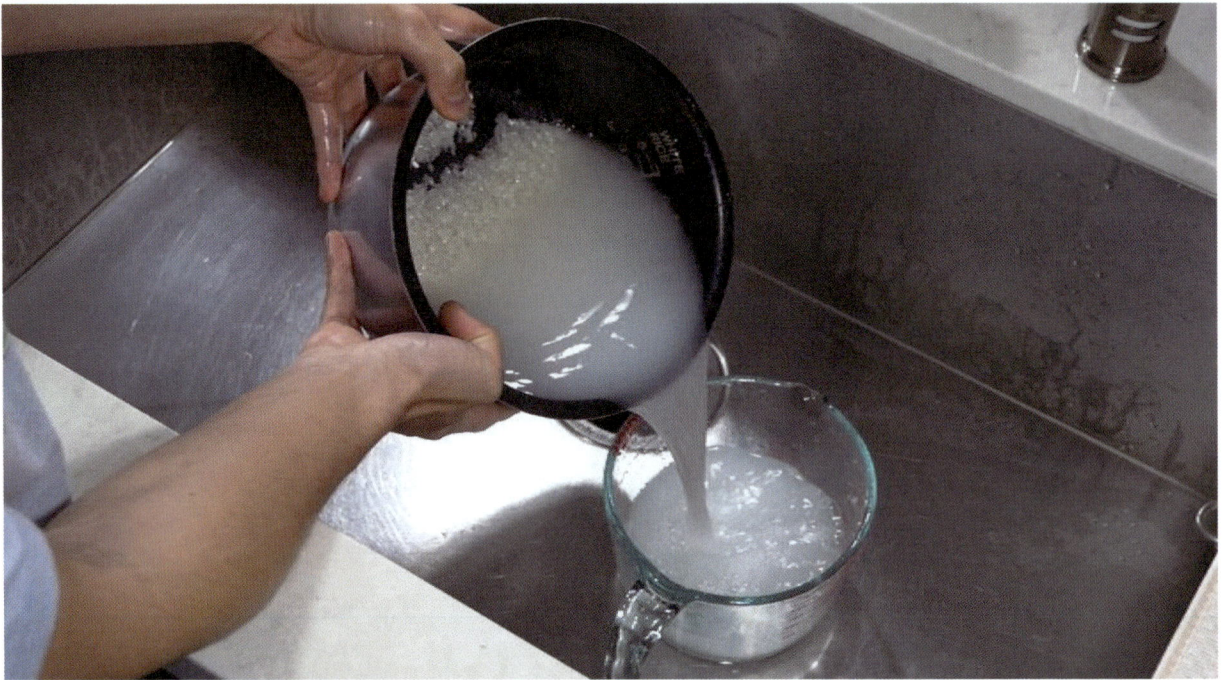

Making togijiru (rice rinse water)

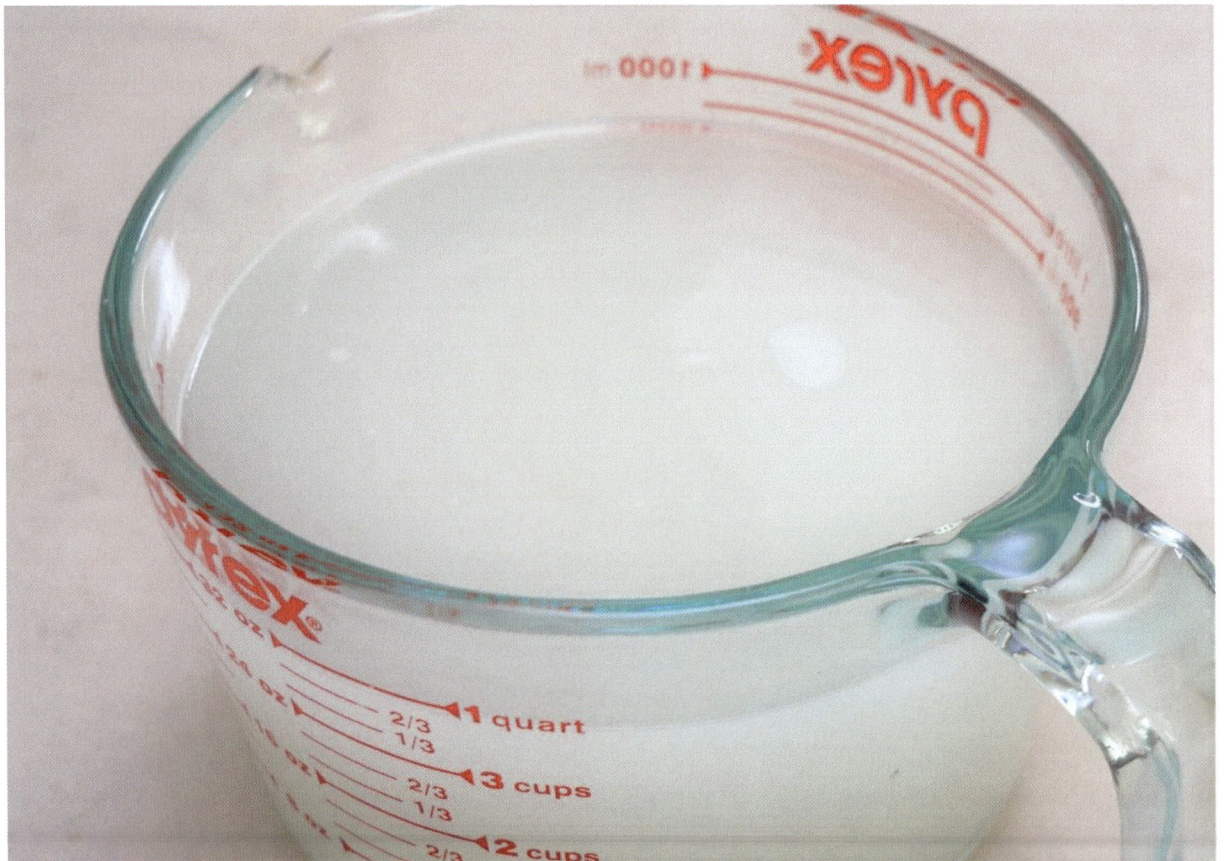

Togijiru (rice rinse water)

Furofuki daikon
(Simmered daikon with sweet miso)
ふろふき大根

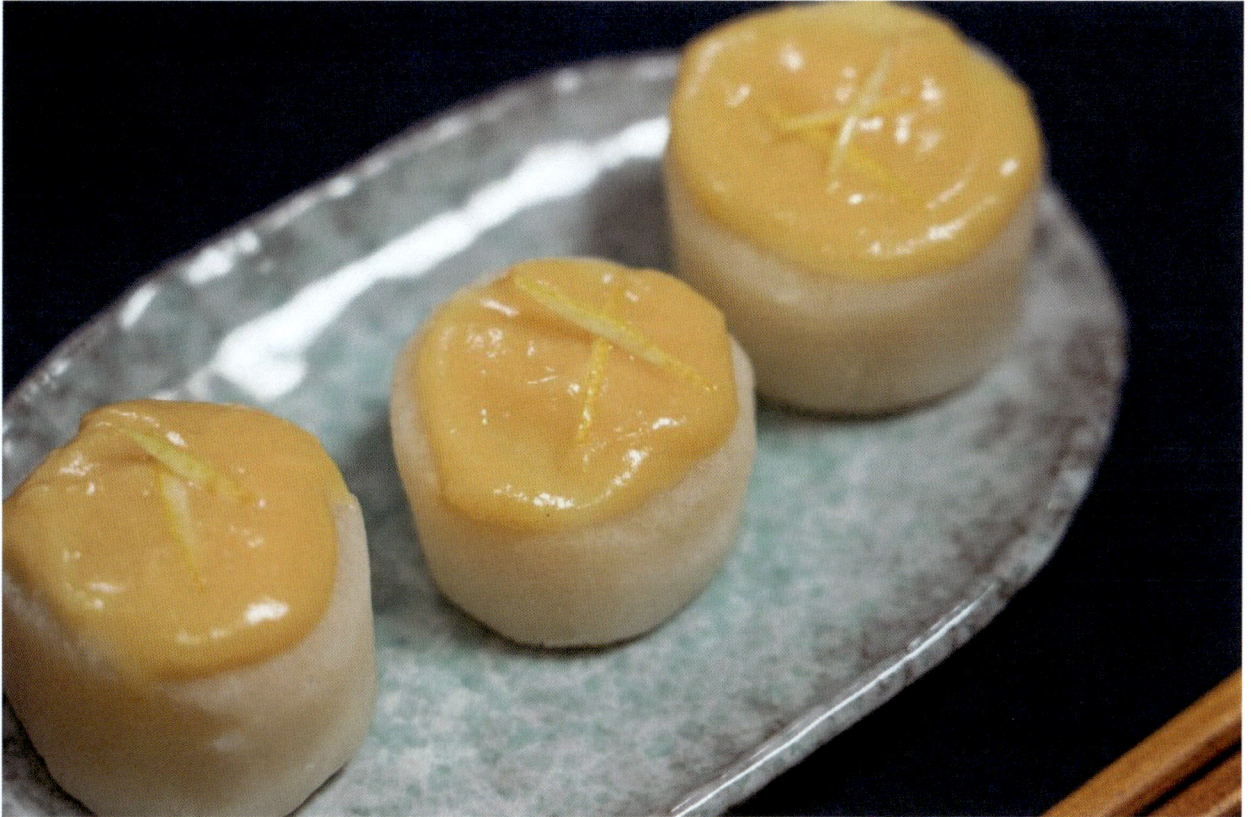

Furofuki daikon could be one of your favorite ways to eat daikon radish. And if you've never had this before, you'll notice the simmered daikon radish has an extremely delicate and pleasant sweetness that's enhanced by the konbu dashi.

This dish is a delicious example of how konbu dashi can make food taste so much better as compared to when it's not used.

The sweet, salty, umami packed miso dengaku sauce is the perfect way to top each piece off.

All you need is some citrus zest to add additional depth and complexity to each bite!

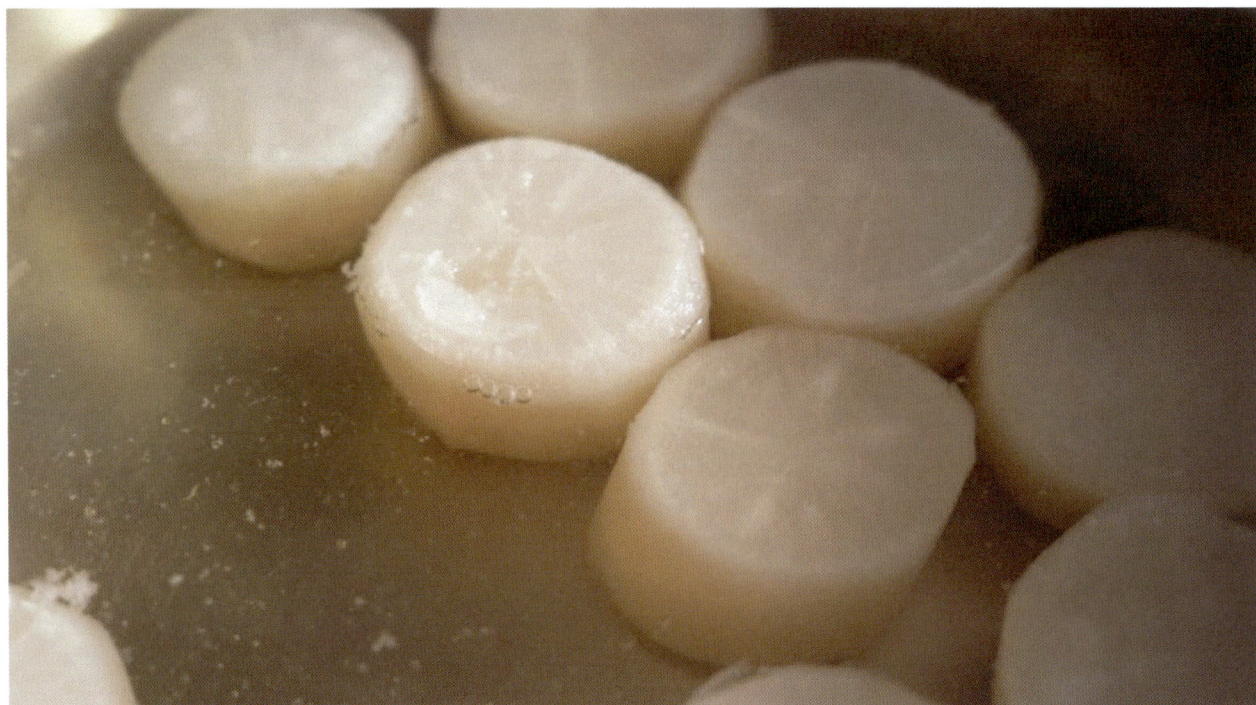

Daikon radish simmering in konbu dashi

Makes 6-8 servings

Ingredients

For the daikon radish

- Two 10-12 in. daikon radishes, peeled and cut 1 in. thick and scored on both sides, mentori* optional
- 6-8 cups togijiru, cloudy white water from rinsing 2 cups of white rice
- 4 cups konbu dashi
- Optional: dash of salt or soy sauce

For the miso dengaku 味噌田楽

- 1 Tbsp sake
- 1 cup mirin
- 3 Tbsps white miso paste
- 2 Tbsps water

Toppings - yuzu, lemon or lime zest

Directions

1. Using a large pot, add the togijiru and daikon pieces and bring to a boil.
2. Simmer for 20-30 minutes until you can pierce the daikon easily with a chopstick.
3. Strain the daikon, discarding the togijiru and return the daikon to the pot.
4. Add in konbu dashi and dash of salt or soy sauce (if using).
5. Simmer with an otoshibuta (or partially covered with lid) for 20-30 minutes.
6. Meanwhile make the dengaku sauce by combining the mirin and sake in a small saucepan. Heat on medium heat and cook until the alcohol has evaporated. Then mix in the miso paste and water. After combined, set aside and allow to cool.
7. Once the daikon has cooked in the konbu dashi, it's ready to serve.
8. Transfer a few pieces to a plate and top generously with miso dengaku and thin slices of zest!

Tips:

- Scoring the daikon on the top and bottom helps to cook the daikon and further infuse the dashi flavor into the flesh. Just press gently with your knife, twice one each side to make a + shape. A ¼ in. deep incision into the flesh is all you need. You can also score other ingredients (such as konnyaku or eggplant) to infuse flavor and expedite the cooking process.
- *Mentori – As mentioned in the kabocha nimono recipe on page 45, this cutting technique helps to preserve the clarity of dashi broth. And though the dashi is not served with the daikon, carving the edges of the daikon pieces does make for a more rounded presentation.
- Avoid boiling the daikon so they maintain their shape, without disintegrating as they soften.
- As with other nimono (simmered dishes), consider using an otoshibuta to maximize the flavor and allow to cool down before eating so that the flavors are fully absorbed.
- Consider using different miso pastes for different flavors of miso dengaku. Red miso pastes tend to be more savory and stronger flavored than white miso pastes which tend to be sweeter.
- You can also use the miso dengaku for other foods like tofu or your favorite vegetables (that have been steamed, grilled, or roasted).
- Consider reusing the leftover konbu dashi for some soup or nabemono (hot pot) such as the mizorenabe recipe found on page 62.

Kanpyou nimono
(Simmered dried bitter gourd)
干瓢煮物

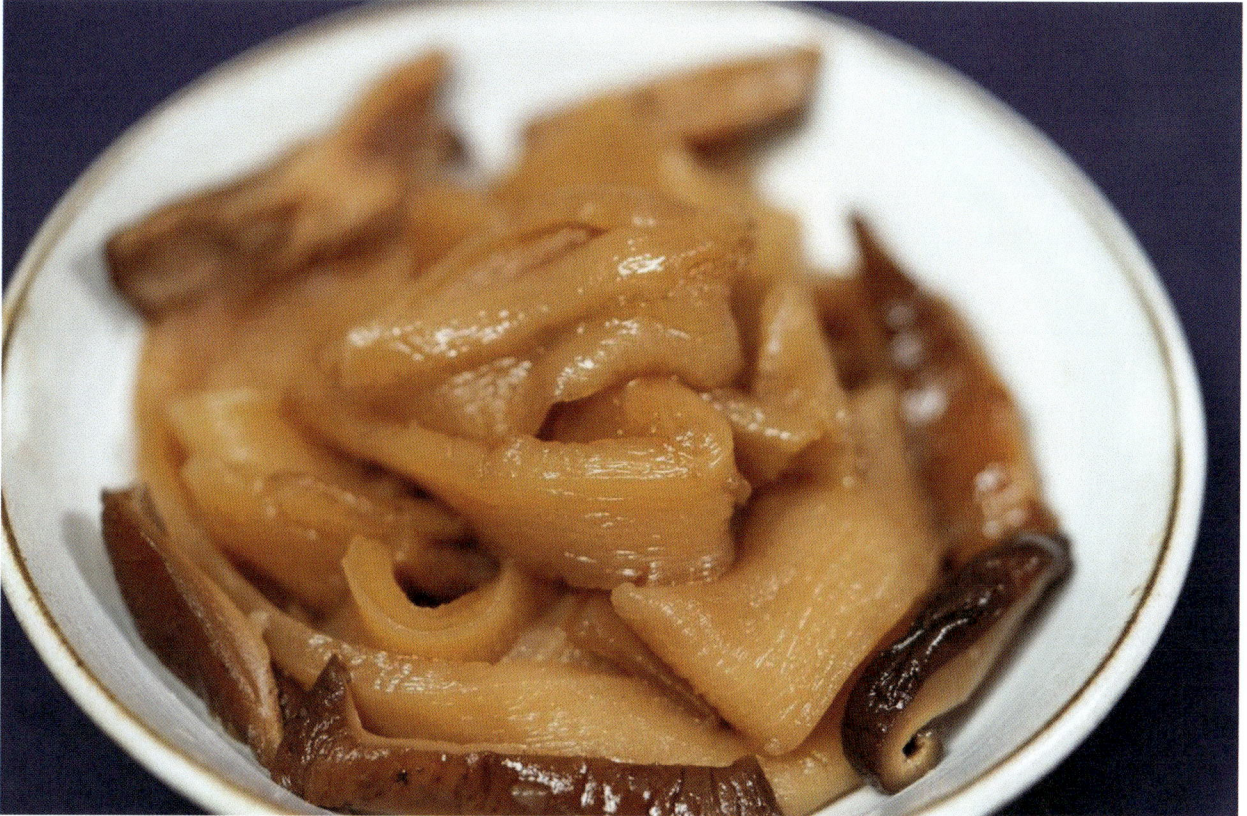

Kanpyou (干瓢 dried bitter gourd) is a dried vegetable that can be used in many different ways.

While this particular dish is meant to be a side dish, you could easily repurpose it for sushi.

For example, in temakizushi (手巻き寿司 handrolls) or makizushi (巻き寿司 cut rolls) or the chirashizushi (ちらし寿司 scattered sushi) recipe found on page 76.

This simmered version also calls for dashigara shiitake (leftover shiitake from making dashi).

So if you've been making a lot of shiitake dashi, this could be a great way to repurpose all the shiitake mushrooms you've saved!

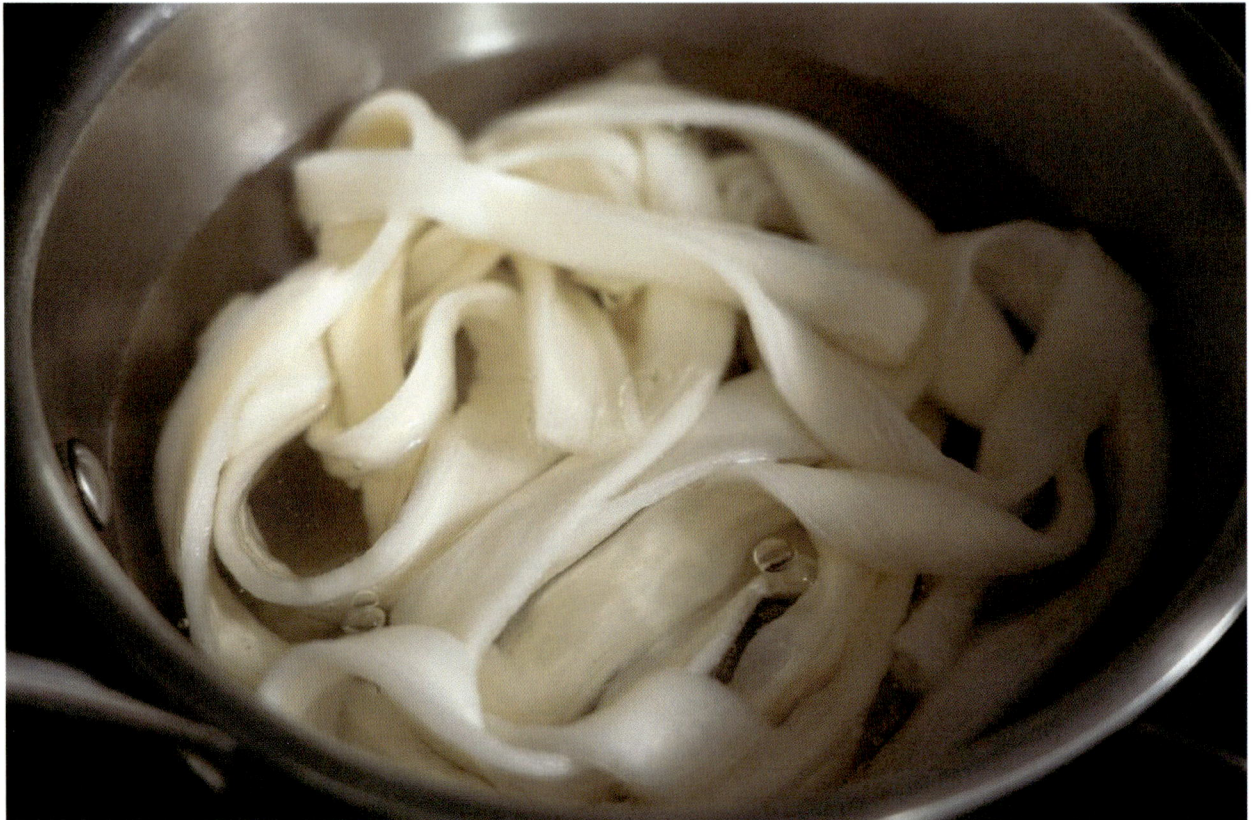

Rehydrated kanpyou

Makes 4–6 servings

Ingredients

- 1 pack dried kanpyou, dried bitter gourd (25-35 g)
- 1 tsp salt
- 3-4 pieces dashigara shiitake, (leftover shiitake from making dashi)
- 1 cup dashi
- 1 ½ Tbsps soy sauce
- 1 ½ Tbsps mirin
- 1 Tbsp sugar

Directions

1. Using a medium sauce pan on medium heat, bring the water to a boil.
2. While the water is heating, rehydrate the dried kanpyou in a bowl with water for about 1 minute.
3. Drain the kanpyou and gently rub pieces together with salt. Add the salted kanpyou to the boiling water and simmer for 10 minutes.
4. Strain the kanpyou. Once cooled, gently press out the excess water.
5. Using a small saucepan, add the dashi with the soy sauce, mirin, sugar, and the kanpyou. Bring to a simmer on medium low heat and cover with an otoshibuta or partially cover with a lid.
6. Once the kanpyou has absorbed all the liquid, remove from heat and serve.

Tips:

- Gently rubbing the kanpyou with salt helps to soften it and aid in rehydration.
- As with other nimono (simmered dishes), consider using an otoshibuta to maximize the flavor and allow to cool down before eating so that the flavors are fully absorbed.
- Consider using raw sugar instead of white sugar for a slightly different flavor.
- Kanpyou nimono will keep for about 3-4 days in the fridge and it freezes well if you want to make a big batch. If freezing, use within three weeks for best flavor.
- You could use all kanpyou or all shiitake mushrooms if you don't have one or the other on hand and adjust the quantity of either accordingly .
- If you prefer a stronger shiitake flavor, use unused dried shiitake and rehydrate them in water for 30 minutes prior to using.

Mizore nabe (Grated daikon hot pot)
霙鍋

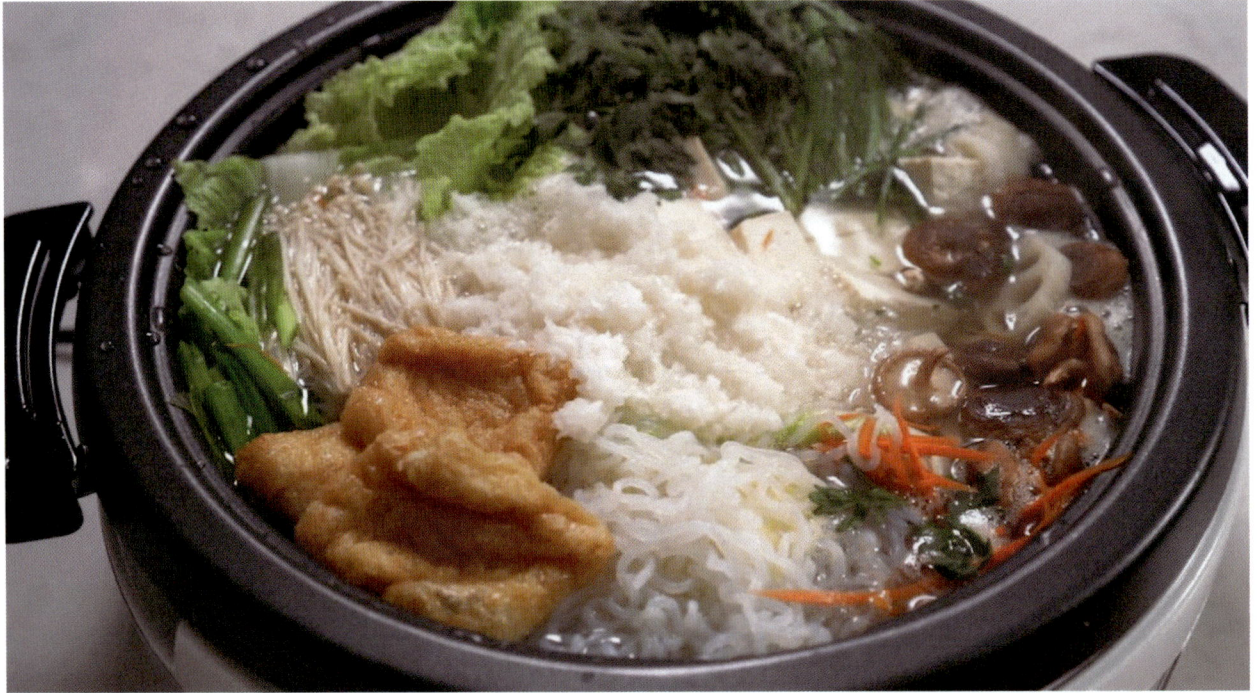

One of the most flavorful ways you can use daikonoroshi is in this mizorenabe. This dish is said to have gotten it's name from the way it looks.

In Japanese, 'mizore' means sleet and 'nabe' is short for nabemono (鍋物 hot pot).

The sharp, pungent, and bitter flavors of the daikon radish mellow out a bit when cooked. Pairing this with the other fresh vegetables and your favorite homemade dipping sauces makes for a very satisfying and filling meal.

Even though nabemono and daikon radish are traditionally winter foods, you could certainly enjoy this anytime of the year.

Makes 4–6 servings

Ingredients

- 4 cups konbu dashi
- ½ cup sake, or mirin (for a slightly sweeter flavor)
- 1 large pack of shirataki noodles, parboiled and cut
- 1 pack aburaage (deep-fried tofu skins), parboiled
- 1-2 blocks firm tofu (14 oz.), drained and cut into small blocks
- ½ bunch shungiku (chrysanethmum greens), chopped into 2-3 in. pieces; alternatively mizuna, bok choy, napa cabbage or cabbage
- 1 cup fresh shiitake mushrooms, sliced
- 1 cup carrots, julienned
- 1 cup renkon, (lotus root) sliced ¼ in. thick
- ½ bunch enoki mushrooms, bottoms trimmed
- 2-3 cups Tokyo negi or green onions, sliced into 1-2 in. pieces
- ¼ cup nira, (garlic chives)
- 2-4 cups freshly grated daikon radish, unpeeled and juices reserved!

Toppings - finely chopped green onion or shiso (perilla), kaiware daikon (radish sprouts), nori (dried toasted seaweed), freshly grated ginger, wasabi, gomashio (ground toasted sesame seeds with salt), ichimi, shichimi or sansho pepper

Dipping sauce suggestions

- Yuzukosho (**柚子胡椒** citrus chili paste) with soy sauce
- Ponzu (**ポン酢** citrus soy sauce)
- nirajouyu (**ニラ醤油** chopped garlic chives with soy sauce)
- umejouyu (**梅醤油** umeboshi with soy sauce)

Directions

1. Add 4 cups of konbu dashi and sake (or mirin) to a large pot.
2. Add in all the vegetables and bring to a simmer.
3. Cover and cook for about 15 minutes until the vegetables and mushrooms are cooked through.
4. Serve with rice and the dipping sauces of your choice!

Tips:

- As mentioned in the kenchinjiru recipe tips on page 39, consider parboiling the aburaage to reduce some of the oil.
- I also recommend parboiling the shirataki noodles, which will not only eliminate the smell, but improve the flavor and texture by reducing some of the water naturally found in the noodles.
- If you can clean and scrub the daikon radish enough to eat without peeling it off, consider grating it that way. Keeping the skin on adds a nice texture once grated. If you decide to peel it, note that the skins can be recycled for use in other dishes like otsukemono (お漬け物 Japanese pickles) or any soup or stew for additional flavor, nutrition, and texture.
- As with any hotpot, you can substitute many of the vegetables. Use whatever is in season. The konbu dashi and sake (or mirin) are packed with umami and naturally enhance all the flavors of the vegetables in this dish.
- I like to keep things organized with the vegetables in their respective areas, but it's up to you how you want to add them to the pot.
- If you're cooking this at the table, you can refill the pot with additional konbu dashi or vegetables as you eat. Save leftover broth to make zousui (雑炊 rice porridge) or mix in a bundle of udon noodles for a different meal!
- Use as much freshly grated daikon as your heart desires and enjoy the refreshing flavors and aroma!

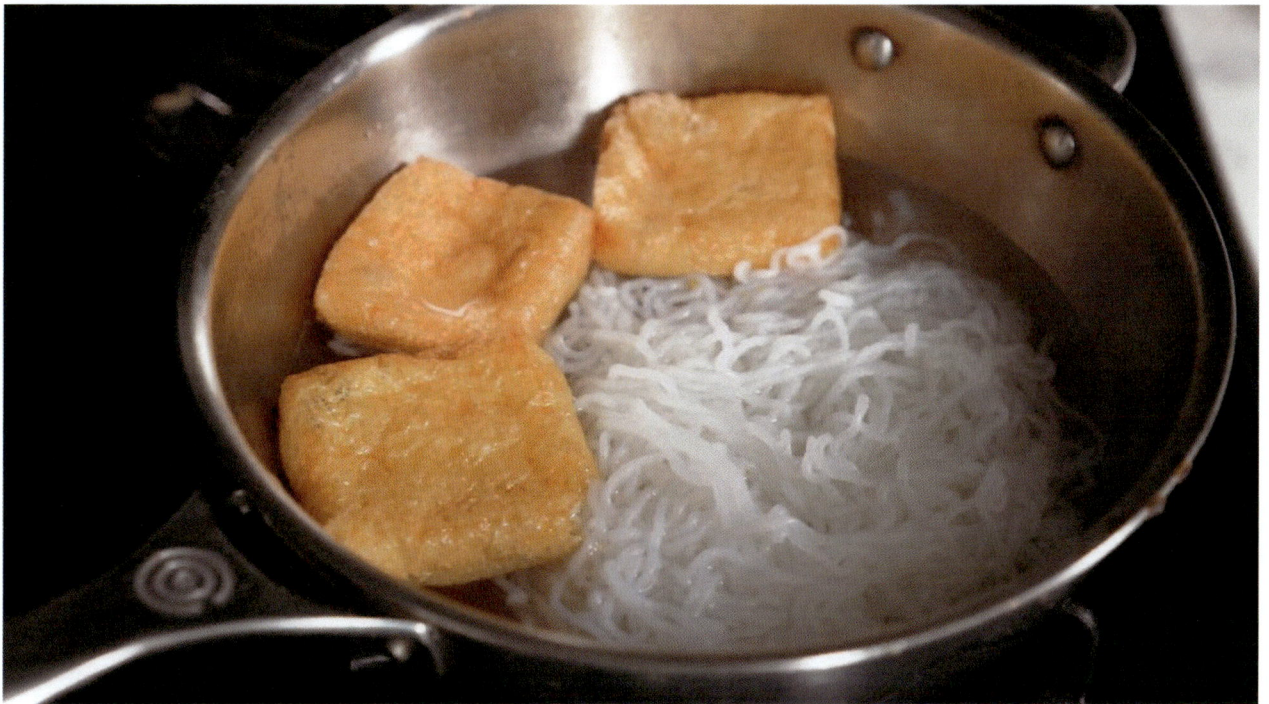

Parboiling aburaage and shirataki noodles

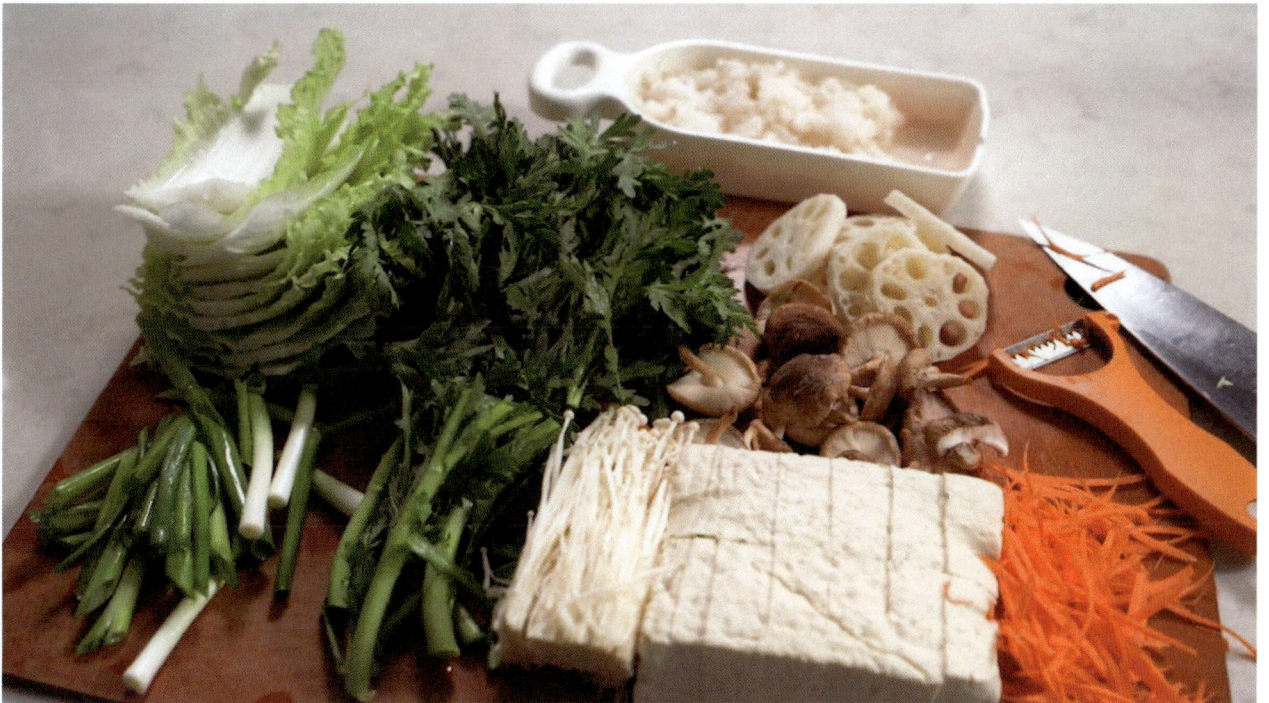

Ingredients for mizorenabe

Goma tounyuunabe
(Sesame soy milk hot pot)
胡麻豆乳鍋

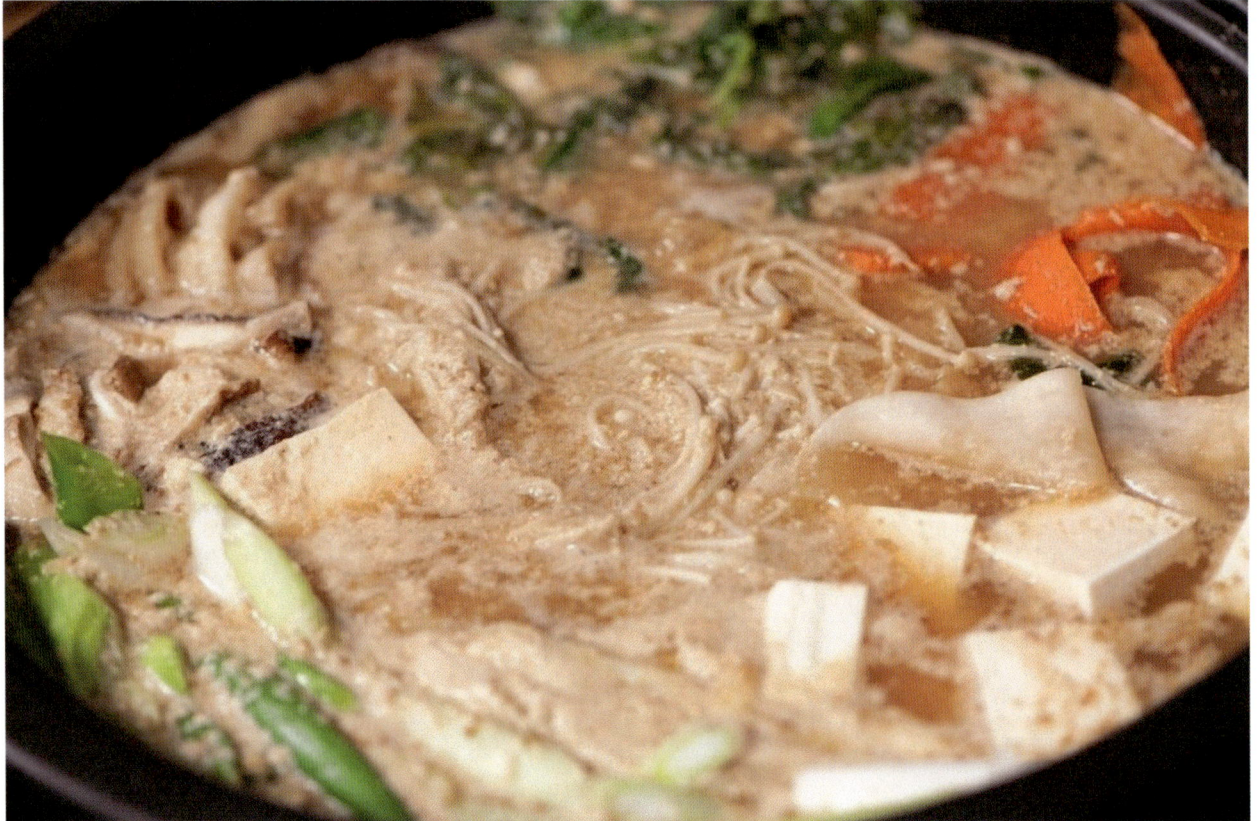

Do you enjoy the flavor of sesame seeds? If so, you're gonna LOVE this hot pot!

The sesame flavor in combination with miso, soy milk and konbu dashi makes for an extremely rich and satisfying meal, possibly unlike any other kind of sesame dish you've ever had.

To make this a complete meal, all you need is a small bowl of rice!

Makes 4–6 servings

Ingredients

- 2 blocks soft tofu (14 oz.), drained and cut into small blocks
- 3-4 cups spinach
- 1 pack enoki mushrooms, bottoms trimmed
- 2-3 cups Tokyo negi or green onions, sliced into 1-2 in. pieces
- 2 cups carrots, thinly sliced (use a mandolin if you have one)
- 2 cups daikon radish, thinly sliced (use a mandolin if you have one)
- 1 cup renkon, (lotus root) cut into half-moon shapes ~1/4 in. thick.
- 1 ½ cups fresh shiitake mushrooms, sliced

For the soup base

- 4 cups konbu dashi
- 3-4 Tbsps red miso paste
- ¼ cup sugar
- 6 Tbsps soy sauce
- ½ cup sesame seeds, toasted and ground
- 2 cups homemade soy milk, thick or regular (thick is double concentrated and will be richer in flavor and texture)

Toppings –sesame seeds (toasted and ground), ichimi or shichimi red pepper

Directions

1. To make the soup base, add 4 cups of konbu dashi to a large pot, along with the miso paste, sugar, soy sauce, and sesame seeds. Stir to dissolve solids and bring to a simmer.
2. Add in the soy milk and all of the vegetables. Start with the root vegetables since they take the longest to cook. *Make sure the vegetables are submerged or if some are not, make sure to turn over halfway through.*
3. Cover and simmer for about 15 minutes until vegetables have softened.
4. Serve with rice and desired toppings.

Tips:

- As with any hotpot dish, you can substitute many of the vegetables and add more as you cook. Just remember the main flavor is going to be sesame. I can't really think of anything that would clash with sesame, but if you think it might maybe test it by using a small quantity of the ingredient first.

Avoid curdling the soy milk broth

- If you're not used to cooking with soy milk, one thing to be mindful of is that it can curdle. Curdling may or may not be an issue for you. If you've never experienced it while cooking, what happens when soy milk curdles is that it separates into a solid portion and liquid portion. Three things that cause soy milk to curdle are: high heat (boiling it), salt (e.g. miso, soy sauce), and acid (e.g. lemon).
- Now that you know there are 3 things that cause soy milk to curdle, here are three ways to reduce the likelihood of curdling it:
  - Avoid boiling the soy milk broth.
  - Add the soy milk just before serving it so it's just heated through.
  - Add a bit of baking soda, ~1/2 teaspoon per cup of soy milk. It will foam so add slowly and carefully to avoid overflowing.

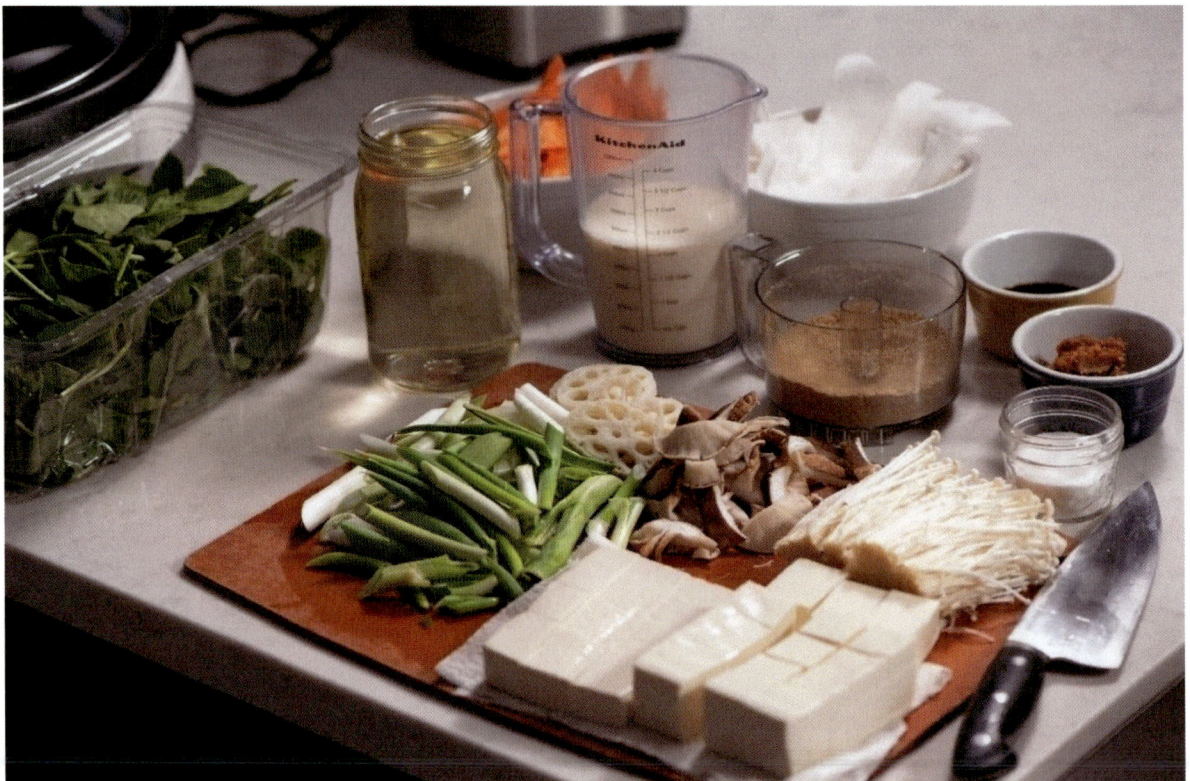

Ingredients for goma tounyuu nabe

Youdoufu (Tofu hot pot) 2 ways
湯豆腐

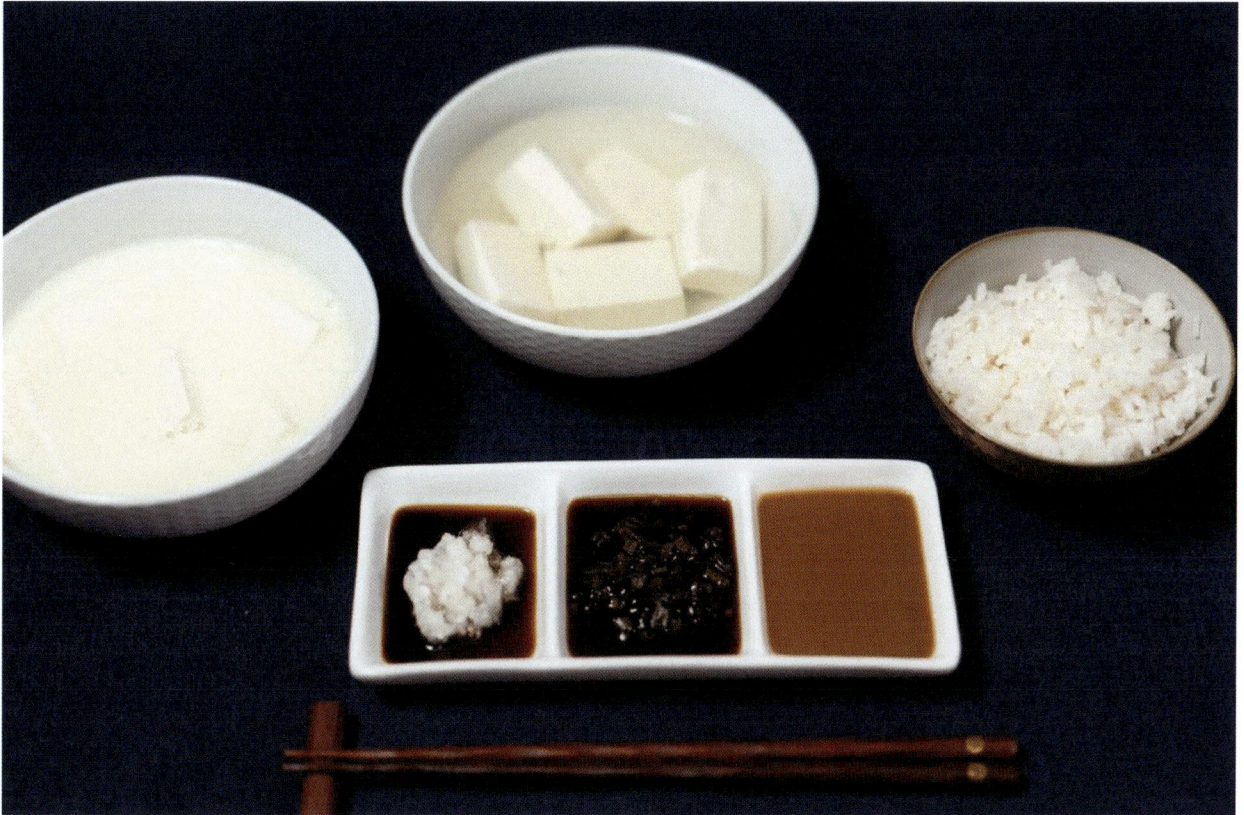

Youdoufu is one of the most simple ways you can enjoy tofu. But don't let that fool you. It's also one of the most delicious, especially when making it at home from scratch. And yes, that includes both the soy milk and the tofu!!

Add in some konbu dashi and/or soy milk, along with a few dipping sauces and toppings, and you'll have a very nice tofu meal.

Just like what you'd find if you were visiting one of the tofu restaurants in Kyoto that specialize in this type of cooking.

Makes 4–6 servings

Ingredients

- 6 cups konbu dashi
- 2 cups homemade soy milk
- 2 blocks homemade tofu; drained and cut into bite-size blocks

Toppings - finely chopped green onion or shiso (perilla), kaiware daikon (radish sprouts), nori (dried toasted seaweed), freshly grated ginger, freshly grated daikon radish, wasabi, gomashio (ground toasted sesame seeds with salt), ichimi, shichimi or sansho pepper

Dipping sauce suggestions

- Yuzukosho (柚子胡椒 citrus chili paste) with soy sauce
- Ponzu (ポン酢 citrus soy sauce)
- Nirajouyu (ニラ醤油 chopped garlic chives with soy sauce)
- Umejouyu (梅醤油 umeboshi with soy sauce)
- Homemade negijouyu (ネギ醤油) see recipe on page 73
- Homemade gomadare (ごまだれ) see recipe on page 73

Directions

1. Add 4 cups of konbu dashi to a large pot. In a separate pot, combine 2 cups soy milk and 2 cups konbu dashi.
2. Add half of the cut tofu to one pot and half to the other. Heat both pots on low heat until they reach a gentle simmer.
3. Use two otoshibuta (drop lids) or partially cover both pots with a lid and cook 15-20 minutes.
4. Serve with rice, dipping sauces, and toppings of your choice.

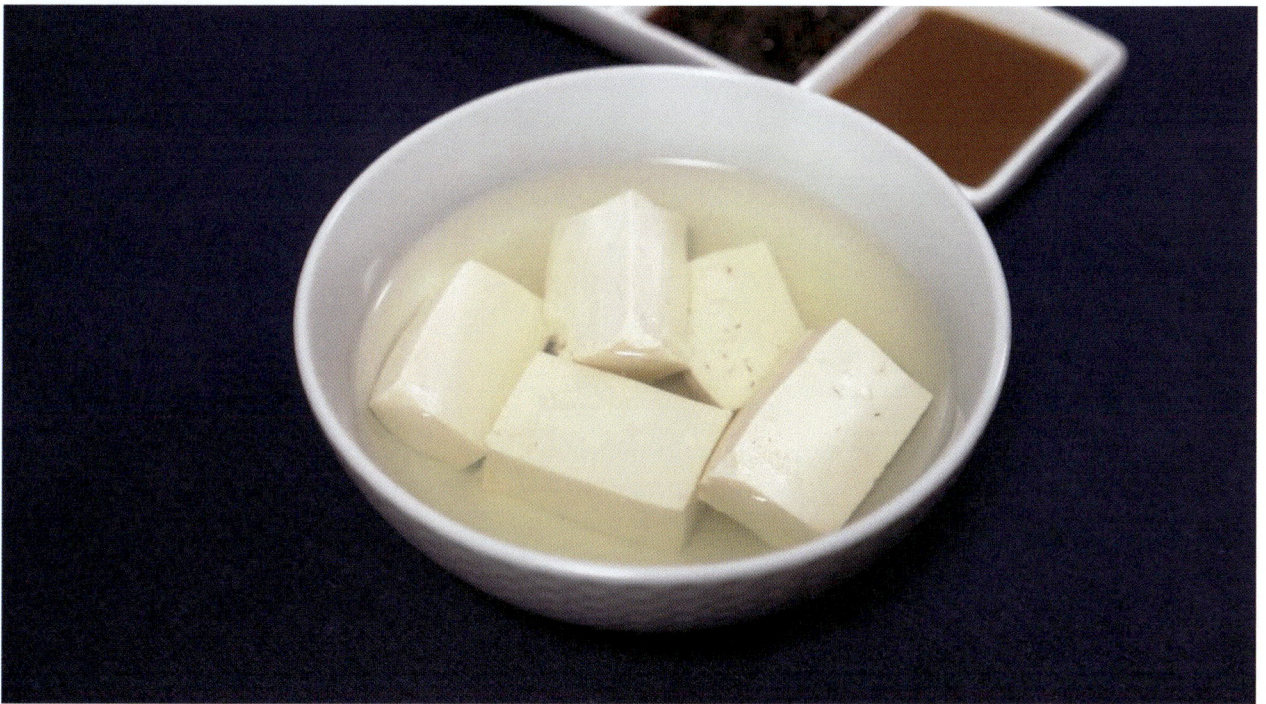

Yudoufu in konbu dashi

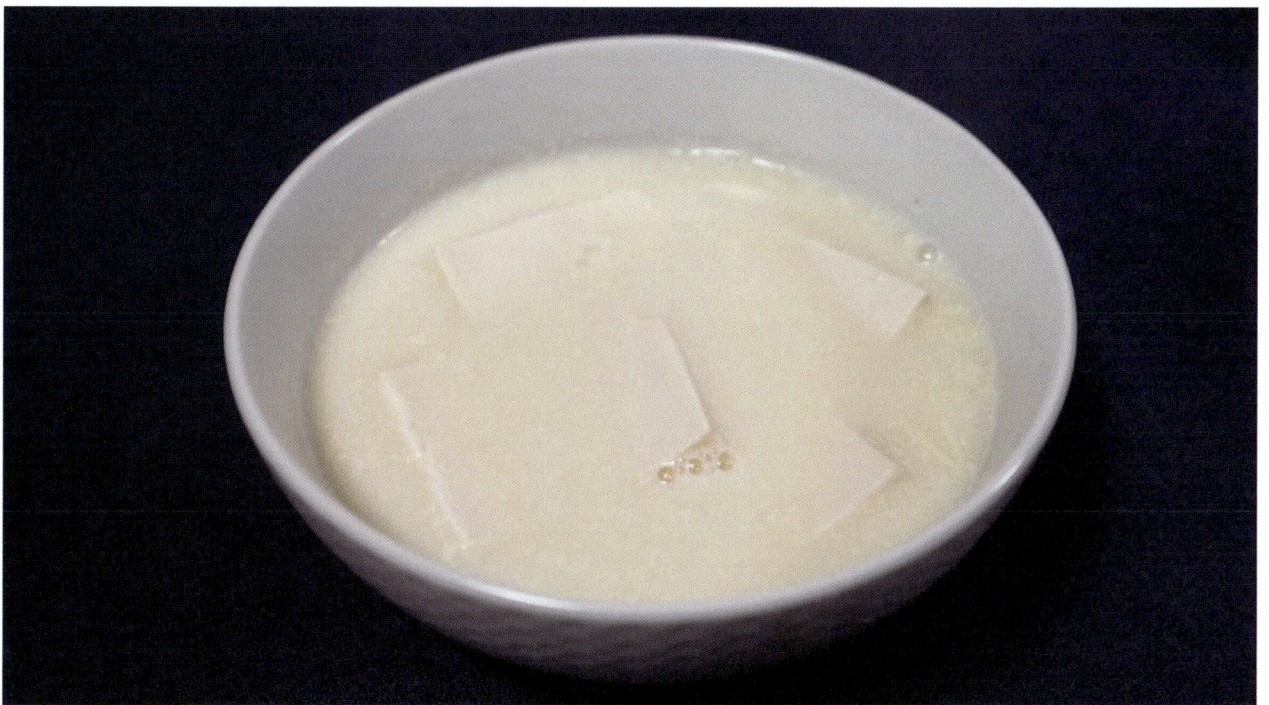

Yudoufu in soy milk konbu dashi

Tips for youdoufu:

- Youdoufu is all about enjoying the natural sweetness and umami of tofu. One of my favorite restaurants in Tokyo is called Ukai. My sister introduced it to me when I was visiting her many years ago. They specialize in tofu and they serve it two ways – konbu dashi and soy milk konbu dashi; just like this recipe! So as you can imagine, this dish brings back many delicious memories from when I was visiting and eating at this and other tofu restaurants in Japan
- When cooking the soy milk dashi mixture, remember to use low heat. This mixture can curdle easily. For more tips on preventing curdling with soy milk, refer to the gomatounyuu nabe recipe tips on page 68.
- If you're using very soft homemade tofu, dropping it into boiling water may cause it to break apart. This is another reason to avoid boiling the youdoufu broth and maintain it at a gentle simmer.
- After you finish cooking the youdoufu, consider saving the broth for a simple nabe (hot pot) the next day. All you need to do is reheat the broth with additional tofu plus any vegetables and you'd like to eat.

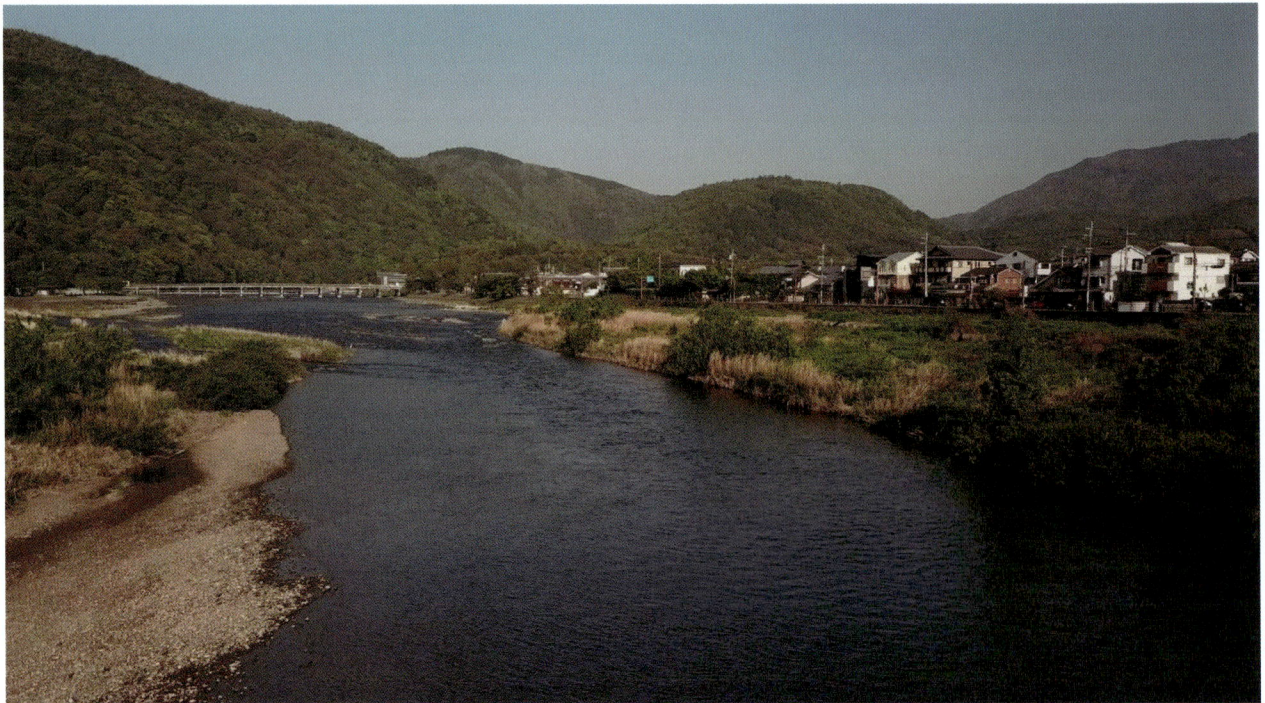

Togestu bridge in the distance, Katsuura River, Kyoto, Japan

Negijouyu (Green onion soy sauce) and Gomadare (Sesame dressing)

ネギ醤油とごまだれ

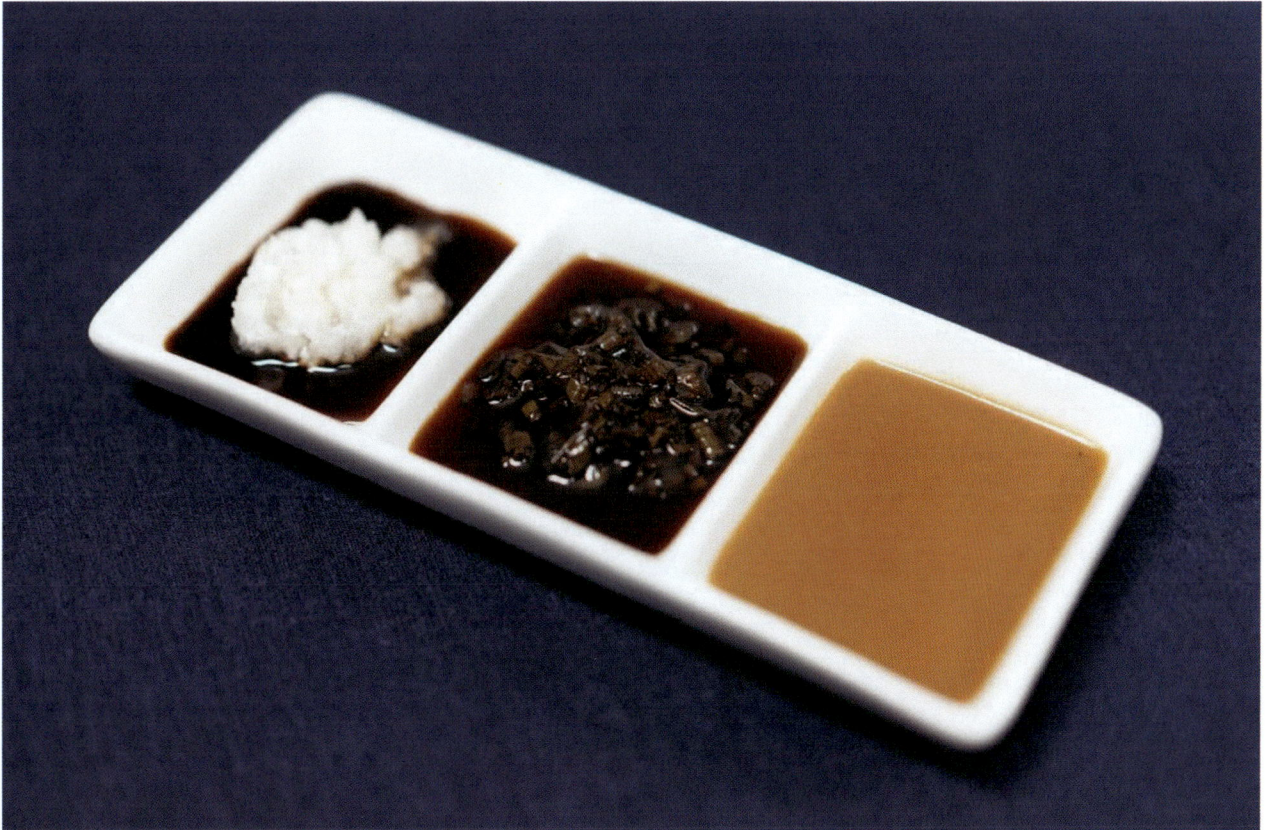

(Left to right) Daikon oroshi in soy sauce, negijouyu, and gomadare

Are you the type of person who enjoys the vehicle (food) more or the sauce that seasons it? Either way, these two dipping sauces might become some of your favorite ways to enjoy nabemono (hot pot).

In spite of calling for just a handful of ingredients, you'll love how bold and flavorful each of these sauces taste. Sometimes simple is all you need!

For the negijouyu (ネギ醤油 green onion soy sauce)

Makes ~ 3/4 cup

Ingredients

- ¼ cup soy sauce
- 2 Tbsps mirin
- 2 Tbsps sake
- ½ cup finely chopped green onion

Directions

1. Combine all ingredients in a small sauce pan and simmer until the alcohol has cooked off. Remove from heat.
2. Serve warm with youdoufu.

For the gomadare (ごまだれ sesame dressing)

Makes ~ 1 cup

Ingredients

- ½ cup sake
- ½ cup mirin
- ¼ cup soy sauce
- 1 Tbsp white miso paste
- ½ cup white nerigoma, (Japanese sesame paste or tahini)
- A few drops of honey or pinches of sugar

Directions

1. Combine the sake, mirin, and soy sauce in a small sauce pan and simmer until the alcohol has cooked off.
2. Whisk together with the remaining ingredients.
3. Serve warm with youdoufu.

Tips for negijouyu and gomadare

- These are both concentrated sauces meant for dipping. However, they can be used for many other things including vegetables, salads, and even soba noodles.
- If you' like a less concentrated seasoning, consider diluting with konbu dashi or water to taste.
- If you have leftovers, refrigerate and use within 3-4 days.

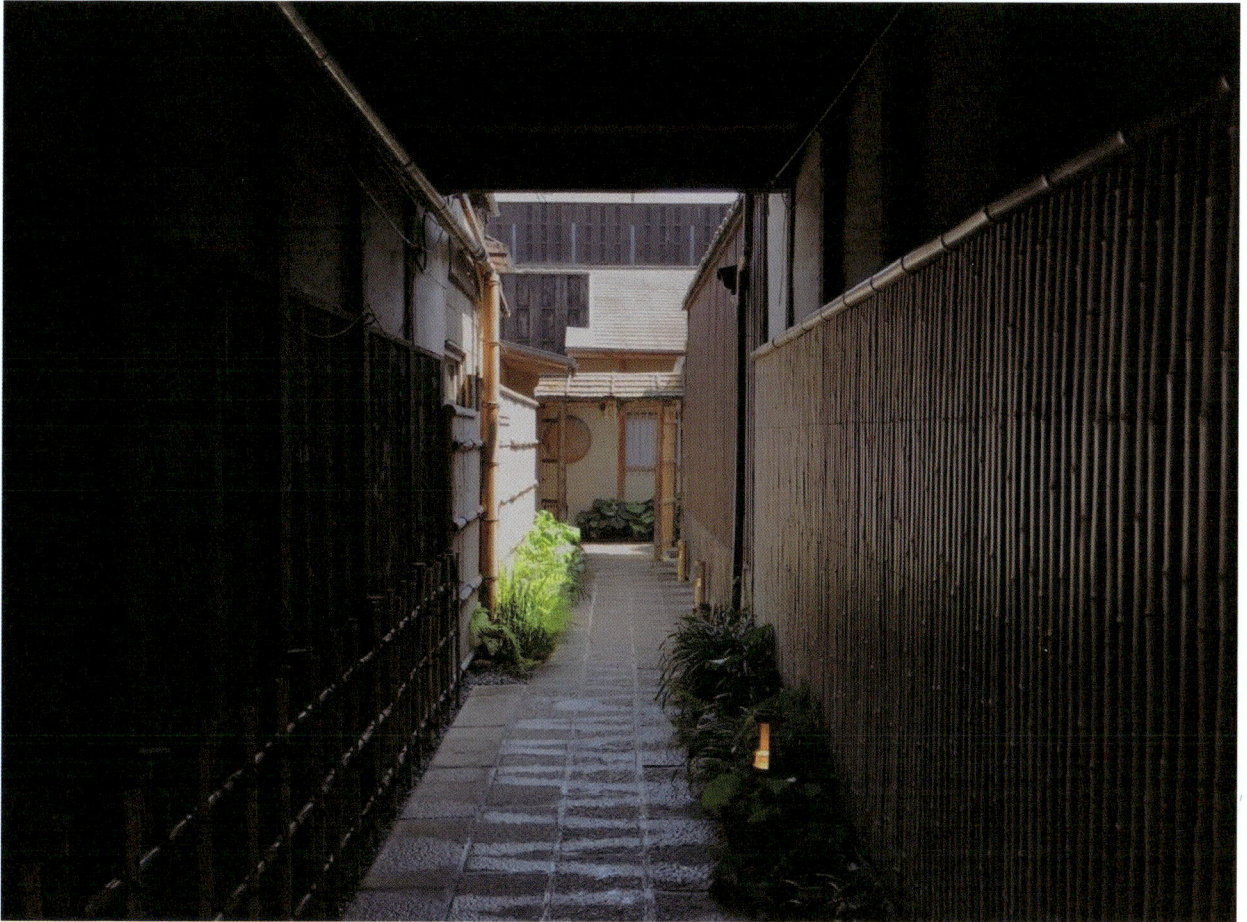

A walkway in the Gion district, Kyoto, Japan

Chirashizushi (Scattered sushi)
ちらし寿司

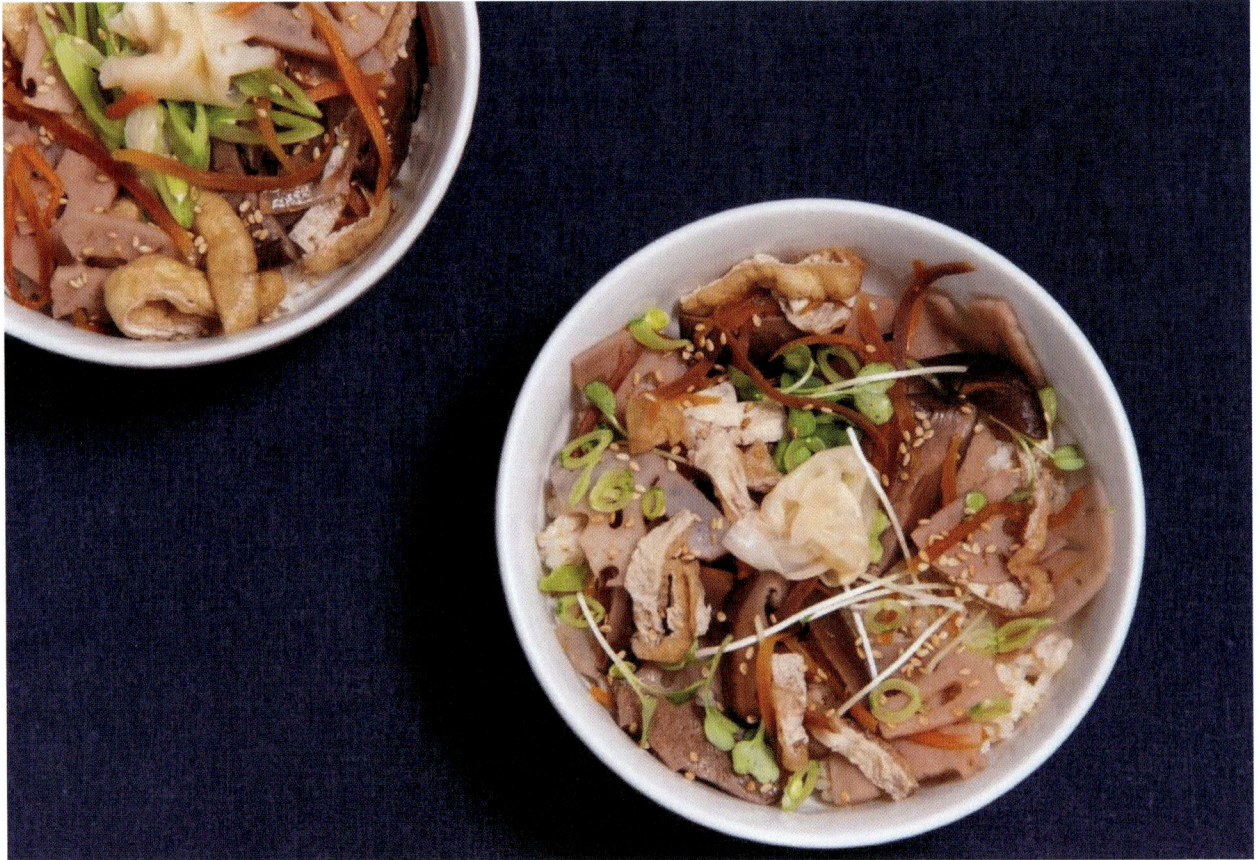

If you've ever tried making makizushi at home, you may appreciate the amount of work it takes to get a perfect and visually appealing sushi roll.

An equally delicious option that requires less work is to skip it all together and make chirashizushi - the easiest type of sushi you can make!

It's packed with delicious flavors, a variety of textures and comes together quite quickly. If you love sushi, you're going to love this chirashizushi.

Makes 4 servings

Ingredients

For the shari (シャリ sushi rice)

- 2 cups Japanese brown rice, (short grain)
- 2 x 2 in. piece of konbu

For seasoning the rice

- 3 Tbsps rice vinegar
- 2 Tbsps sugar
- 1 tsp salt
- Optional: 2 Tbsps white sesame seeds, toasted

For the vegetables

- 1 cup dashi
- 1 Tbsp light soy sauce, (usukuchi shouyu)
- 1 Tbsp mirin
- ½ Tbsp sugar
- 2-3 large pieces aburaage, (deep fried tofu skins), thinly sliced
- 1 cup carrots, julienned
- 1 cup renkon, (lotus root) thinly sliced and cut into quarters
- 8 fresh shiitake mushrooms or dashigara (leftover shiitake from making dashi)

Toppings -1 cup of snow or sugar snap peas (sliced thinly at an angle), pickled ginger, wasabi, kaiware daikon (radish sprouts), nori (dried seaweed)

Directions

To make the shari

1. Cook the rice in your rice cooker with konbu (which helps improve the flavor).
2. Meanwhile, mix the rice vinegar, salt, and sugar and microwave for 20-30 seconds to dissolve. Stir to dissolve any remaining salt or sugar crystals and set aside.

3. Once the rice is done, gently fold in the rice vinegar mixture (and sesame seeds if using) .
4. Allow rice to cool to room temperature.

To make the vegetables

1. Using a small sauce pan add the dashi, light soy sauce, mirin and sugar and bring to a simmer.
2. Add the carrots, shiitake, renkon, and aburaage. Cook for 15 minutes stirring occasionally, until most of the liquid has reduced.
3. Allow to cool to room temperature.

To serve

1. Layer 1 to 1 ½ cups brown sushi rice to the bottom of a bowl.
2. Scatter the vegetables on top, followed by your desired toppings, and enjoy!

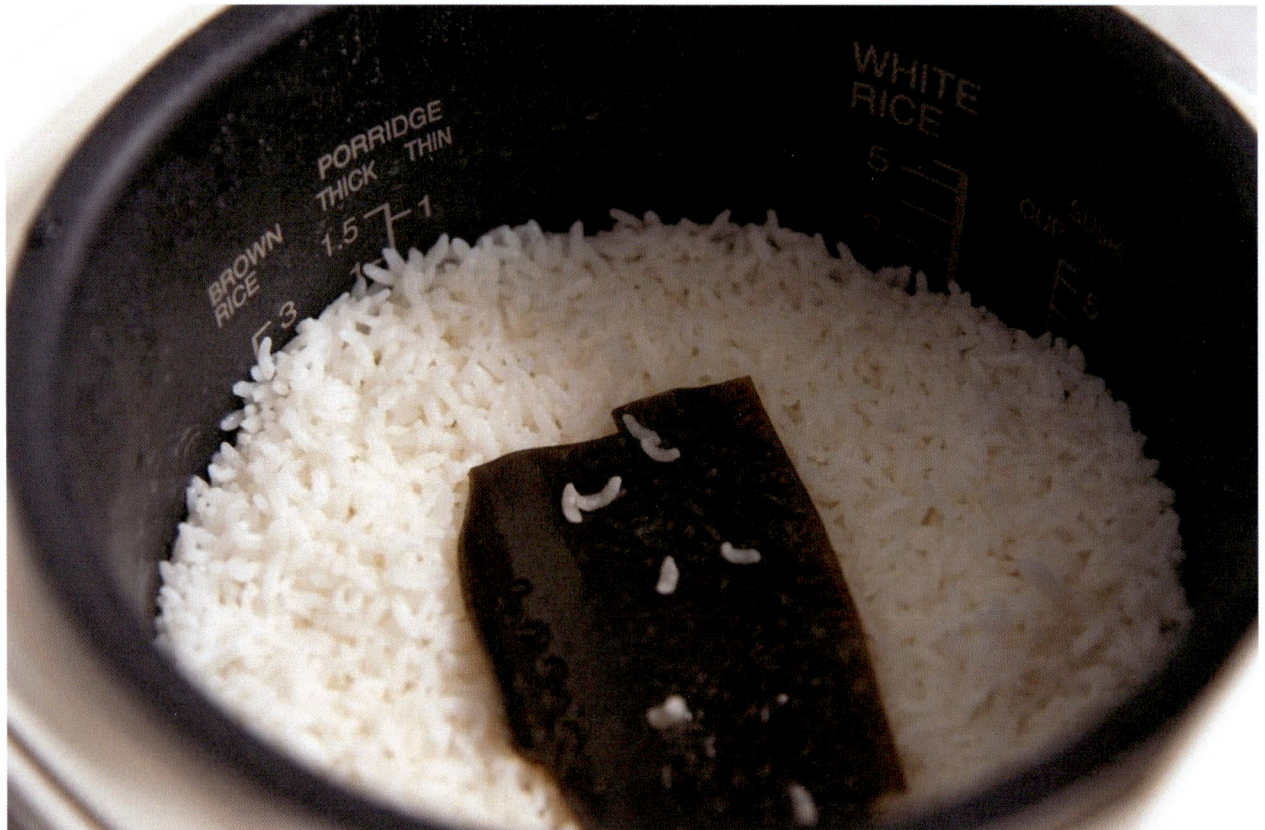

Cooked white rice with konbu

Tips:

- Substitute the vegetables to suit your tastes. Try using thinly sliced and sautéed bell peppers or eggplant, green beans, and thin strips of tofu. Cucumber and avocado are also a nice addition. If you feel you need additional seasoning, consider using a few dashes of soy sauce.
- After you mix the sweet vinegar with the rice, fan the rice to speed cooling and improve the texture (to avoid mushy rice).
- Consider mixing the sesame seeds into the rice instead of scattering on top.
- Instead of cooking the aburaage with the vegetables, try lightly toasting it with a bit of salt for a crunchy texture.
- If you prefer a non-fried tofu alternative, use tofu that's been drained and broiled for a few minutes on both sides (to give it a nice crust).
- If you don't want to make the sushi vinegar from scratch – you have a couple of options:
  - Sushinoko (**すしのこ** powdered sushi seasoning) or bottled sushizu (**すし酢** sushi vinegar made with sugar instead of corn syrup if possible).

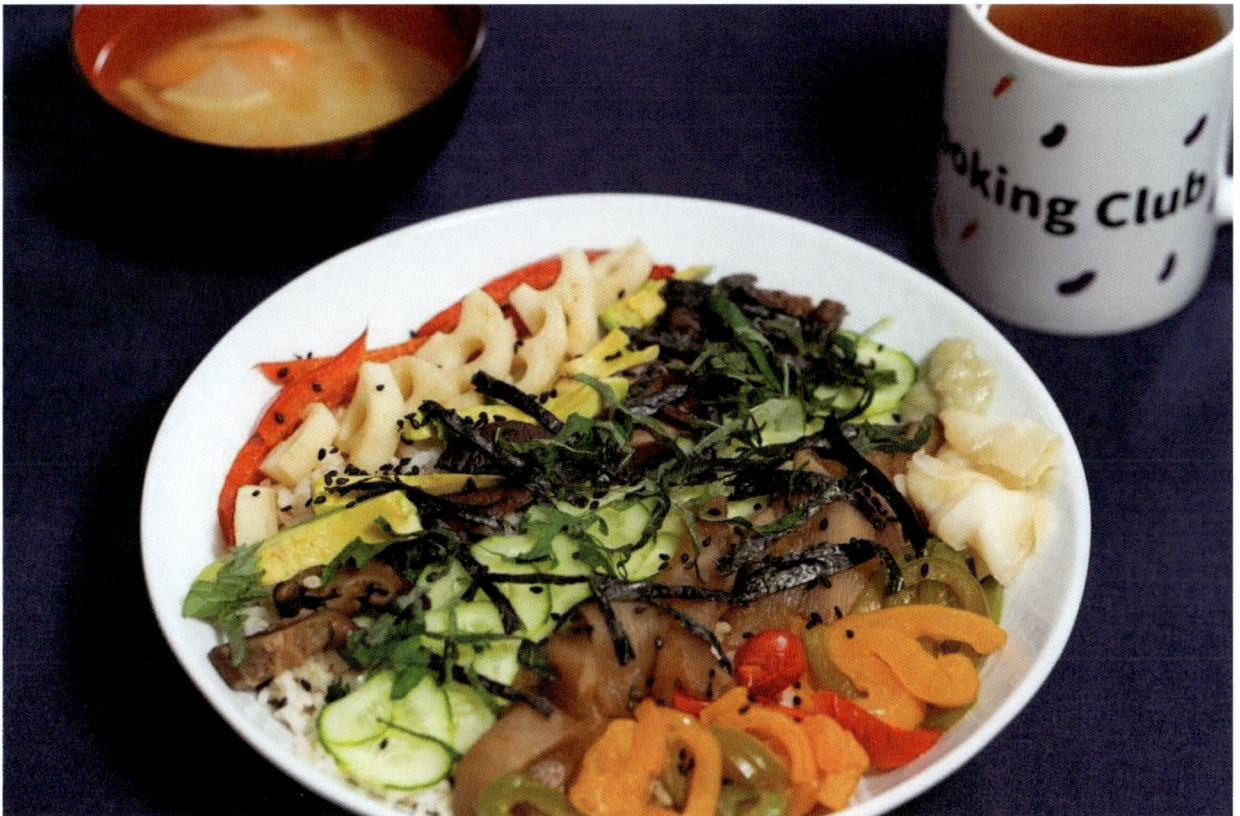

Chirashizushi with peppers, renkon, avocado, shiitake, cucumber, kanpyou nimono, and pickled ginger

Yasai ankakedonburi (Vegetable rice bowl)
野菜丼

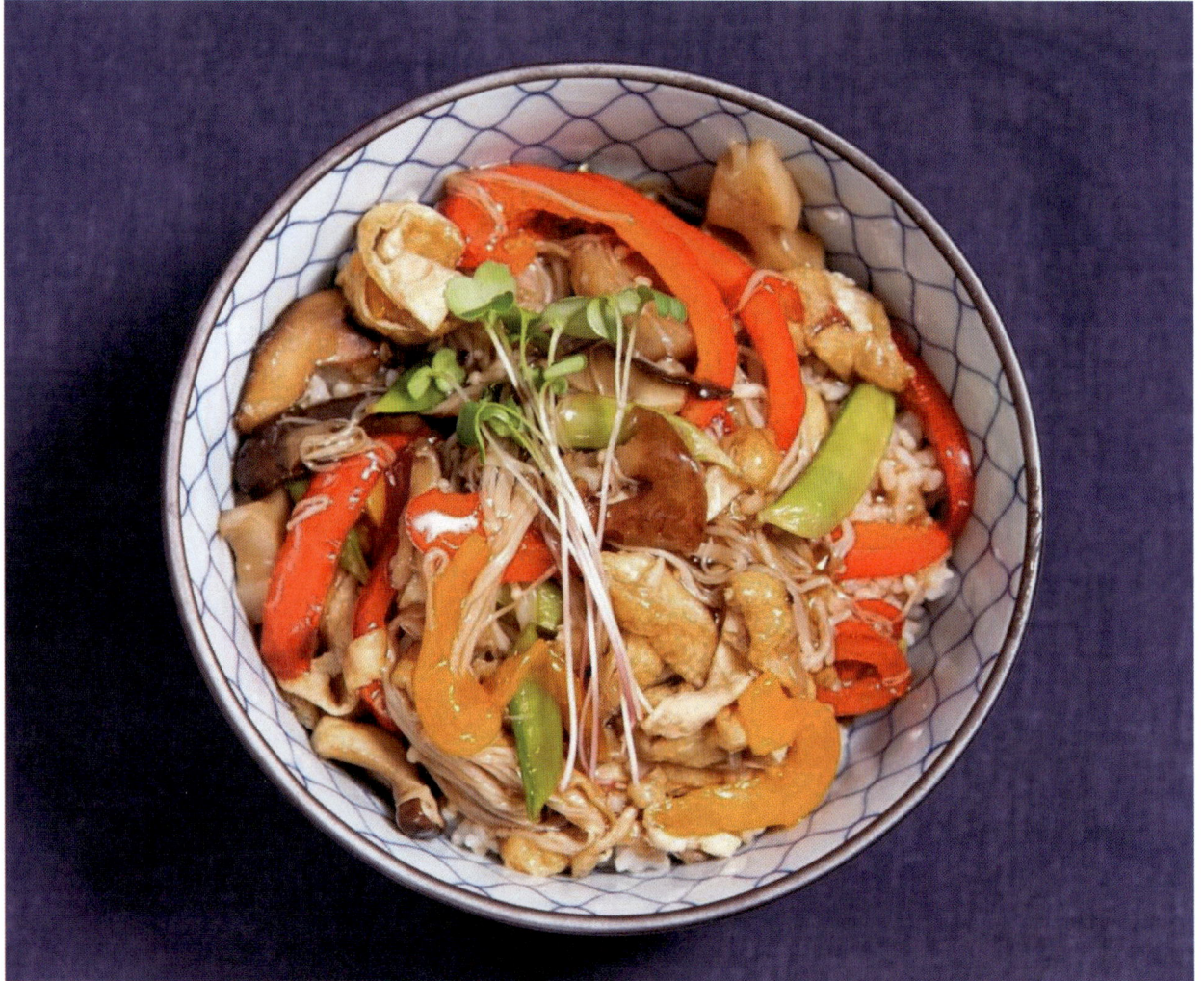

Love a good rice bowl? If not, let this be your first!

This could be your new favorite one-dish meal, full of flavor, color and nutrition. This has been on my rotation for years because it's not only simple to make, but tastes delicious too!

Makes 2-3 servings

Ingredients

For the an (あん sauce)

- 2 cups shiitake dashi
- 2 Tbsps mirin, nikkitta (microwaved 20-30 secs to evaporate the alcohol)
- 2 Tbsps light soy sauce, (usukuchi shoyu)
- 1 ½ Tbsps potato starch in 3 Tbsps water

For the vegetables

- 1 cup renkon, (lotus root) sliced ¼ in. thick and quartered
- 1 ½ cups fresh shiitake mushrooms, sliced ¼ in. thick
- 2 pieces aburaage (fried tofu skin) or small strips of firm tofu
- ¼ red bell pepper, sliced ¼ in. thick
- ¼ yellow bell pepper, sliced ¼ in. thick
- ½ cup snow or sugar snap peas
- ½ bunch enoki mushrooms, bottom trimmed
- 1-2 Tbsps Extra virgin olive oil, or sesame oil

For serving

- Japanese brown rice (short grain) or udon noodles

Toppings - kaiware daikon (radish sprouts), shiso (perilla), chopped green onions, white pepper, ichimi or shichimi red pepper

Directions

To make the an sauce

1. Add the shiitake dashi, mirin, and light soy sauce to a small saucepan and heat to a gentle simmer.
2. Get the potato starch slurry ready by stirring it to eliminate any clumps.
3. Gradually add the potato starch slurry into the dashi mixture stirring continuously to avoid clumping. Bring to a gentle boil and within a minute or so, the mixture should be noticeably thicker.
4. Once thickened, remove from heat and cover.

To make the vegetables

1. Using a large pan on medium heat, add the oil and cook the renkon and mushrooms for 1-2 minutes.
2. Add in the rest of the vegetables and cook for 4-5 minutes until softened. Stir occasionally, allowing them to brown slightly.
3. Once the vegetables have softened, add all the 'an' sauce to the vegetable pan and mix the vegetables into the sauce.
4. Remove from heat.

To serve

1. Place one serving of brown rice into a bowl and pour the vegetable 'an' sauce over the rice. Use one generous cup of rice (or 1 bundle of udon noodles) and one generous cup of vegetables with an sauce per person.
2. Top with desired toppings and enjoy!

Tips:

- Other vegetables that work well in this dish are onion, shredded carrots, okra, baby corn, bamboo shoots, eggplant, zucchini, tomatoes, spinach or mizuna. Basically anything that you'd use in a stir fry would go well with the 'an' sauce.
- Use any leftover vegetable 'an' sauce as a side dish on it's own or to season other foods such as a block tofu.

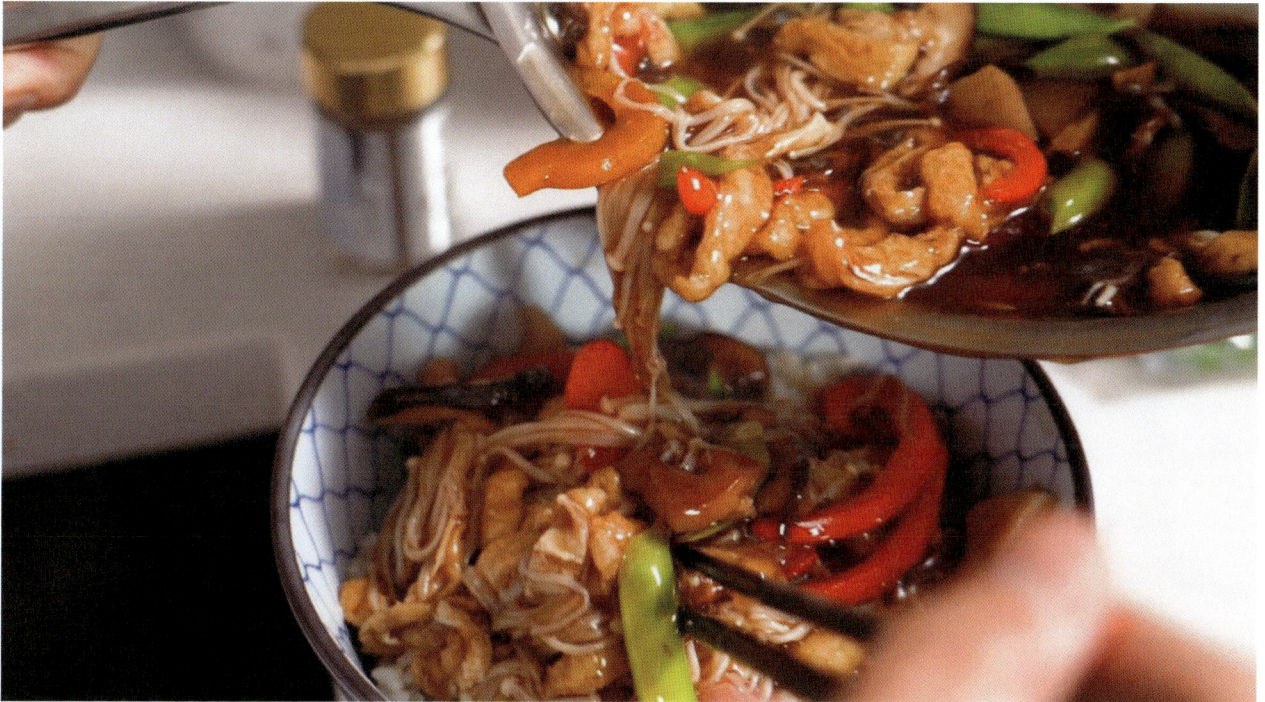

Pouring the vegetable 'an' sauce on top of brown rice

Inarizushi (Stuffed marinated tofu skins)
いなりずし

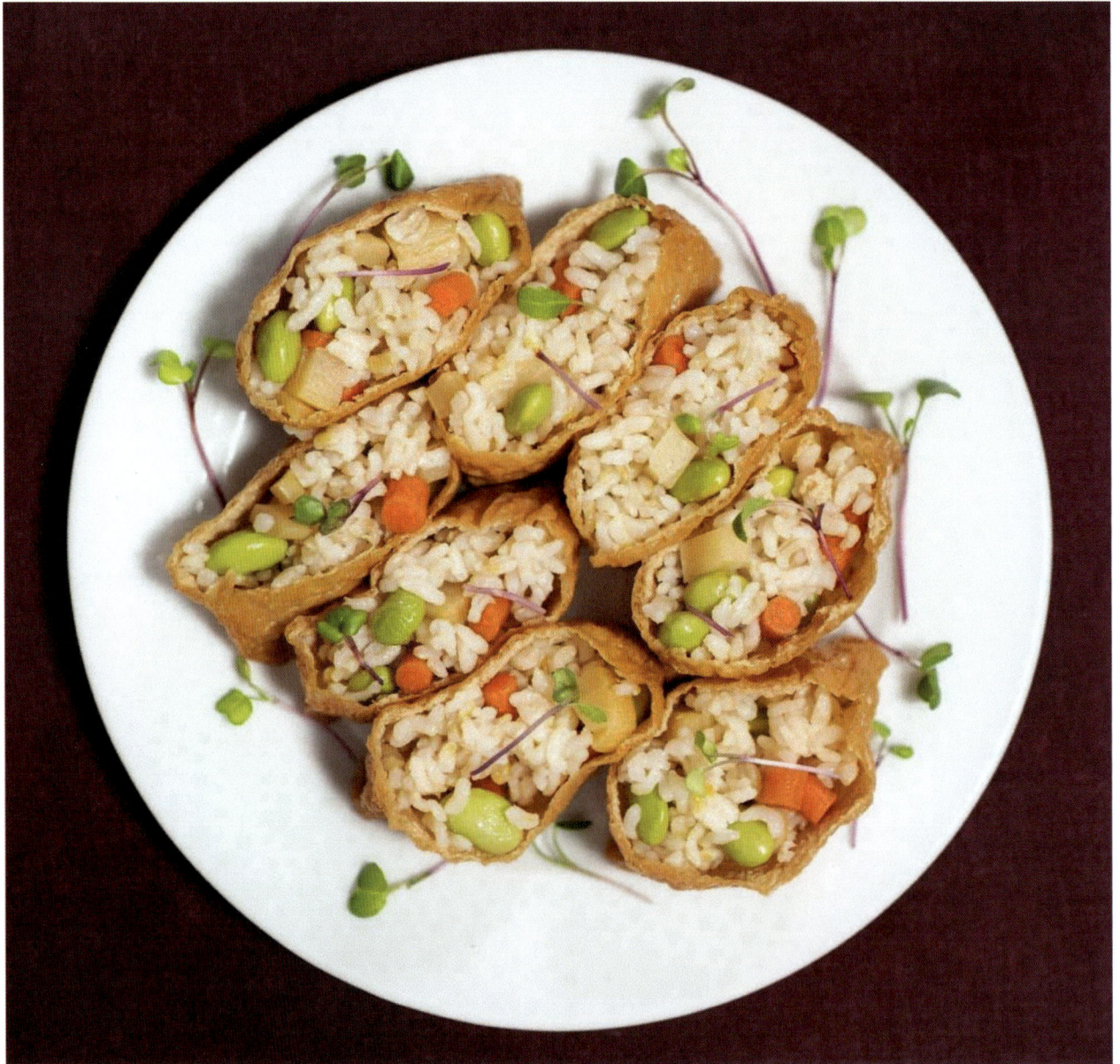

Growing up, this was one of my favorite things to eat on New Year's Day!

Inarizushi is full of flavor and has no fish! (which I didn't like when I was little).

This take on traditional inarizushi takes the base flavors a step further with a few different textures, flavors and colors.

Brown rice helps to make each piece more nutritious and filling.

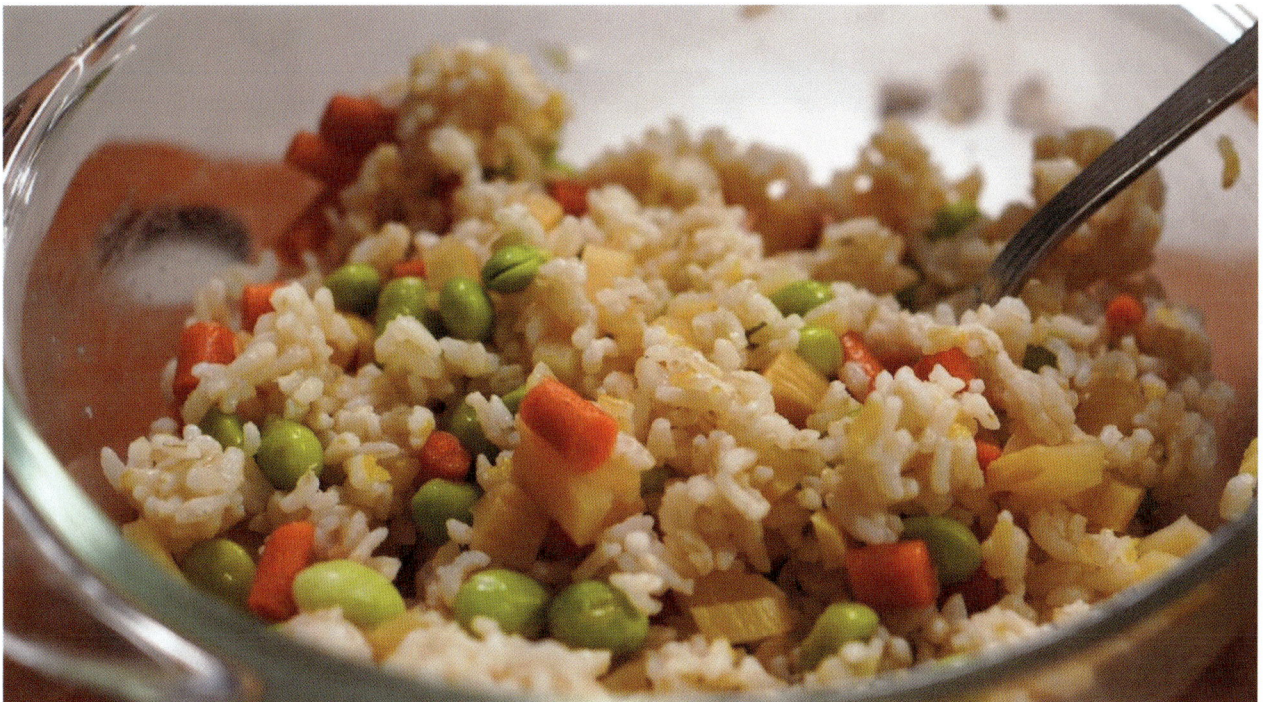

Filling for the inarizushi

Makes 4-6 servings

Ingredients

For the shari (シャリ sushi rice)

- 2 cups Japanese brown rice, (short grain)
- 2 x 2 in. piece of konbu

For seasoning the rice

- 3 Tbsps rice vinegar
- 2 Tbsps sugar
- 1 tsp salt

For the vegetables

- 1 pack of inari, (fried and marinated tofu pouches)
- ½ cup takuan, (pickled daikon radish) cubed
- ½ cup pickled gobo (burdock root) cubed
- ½ cup edamame, boiled in salted water and shelled

Toppings: kaiware daikon (radish sprouts), pickled ginger, toasted sesame seeds

Directions

To make the shari

1. Cook the rice in your rice cooker with konbu (which helps improve the flavor).
2. Meanwhile, mix the rice vinegar, salt, and sugar and microwave for 20-30 seconds to dissolve. Stir to dissolve any remaining salt or sugar crystals and set aside.
3. Once the rice is done, gently fold in the rice vinegar mixture.
4. Allow to cool to room temperature and then mix in the cubed vegetables.

To assemble the inarizushi

1. Gently squeeze the marinade out of the pouches (unless you like them juicy).
2. Use a spoon or fork to fill each pouch with the rice vegetable mixture until full.
3. Holding the stuffed pouch in one hand, press the rice filling down firmly with two fingers.
4. Repeat until all the rice or pouches have been used.
5. Serve immediately.

Tips:

- If you can't find pickled gobo, use cubed carrots (boiled, drained and soaked in rice vinegar for at least 20 minutes). Another alternative is cubed bell pepper (red, yellow, and orange), also soaked in rice vinegar for about 20 minutes. For the green color, you can use green peas, sugar snap peas or avocado!
- The tofu pouches can vary in size, but 1 pouch holds about ¼ cup cooked rice.
- The inarizushi liquid that the tofu pouches come in is full of flavor. Try adding some to the rice and see if you like the additional salty/sweet flavor.
- Leftover pouches can be frozen for up to three weeks in an airtight ziplock or glass container.

Yubadonburi (Tofu skin rice bowl)
湯葉あんかけ丼

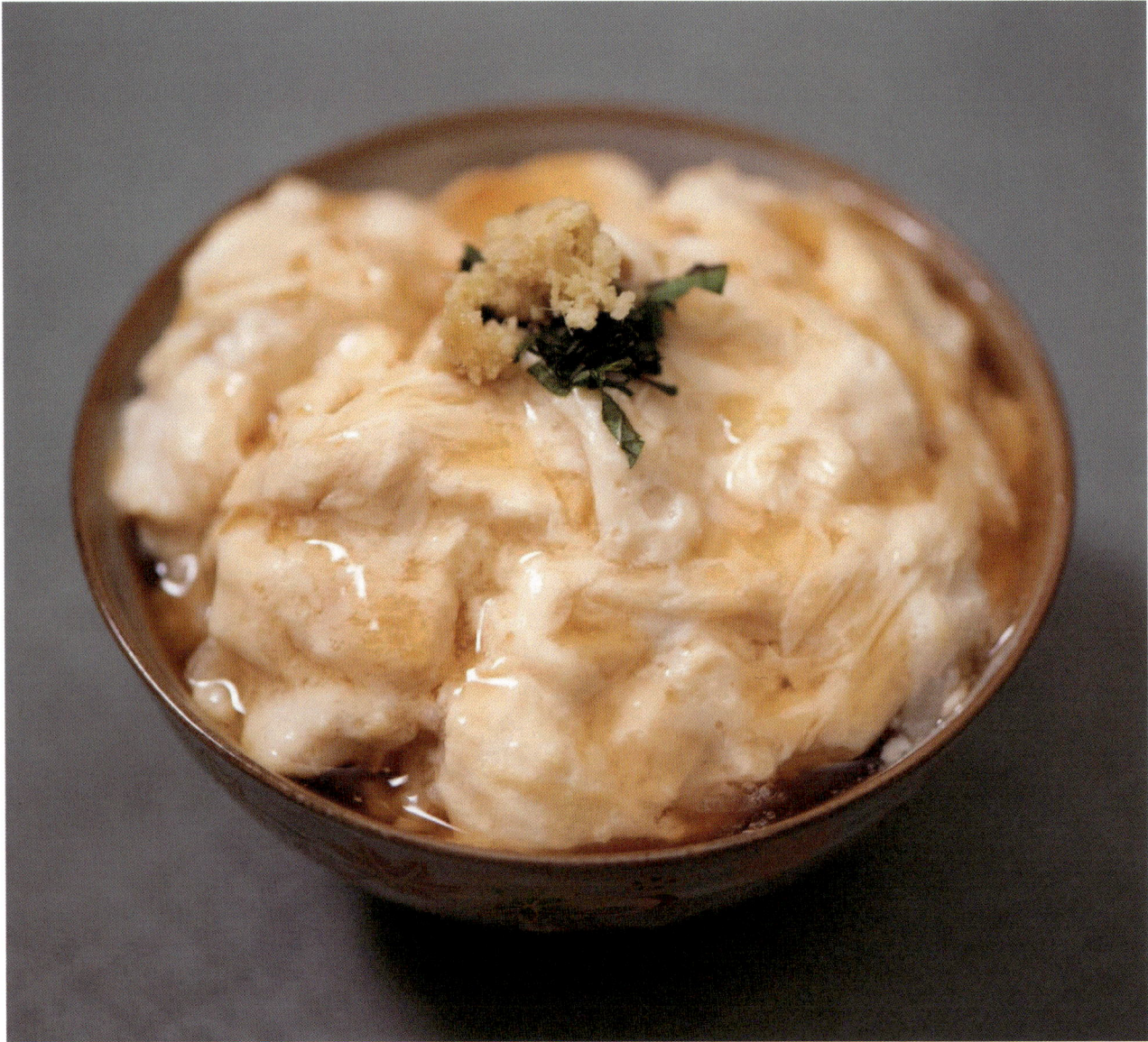

Yuba is one of my favorite soy products. I consider it quite a delicacy. Like toro (トロ fatty tuna) is to tuna, I feel like yuba is to soy. It does take a while to make at home but the resulting flavor and textures are mind-blowing!!

I always make a large batch of yuba using several burners and pans. After finishing, I save the leftovers in soy milk overnight. It's just as good the next day!

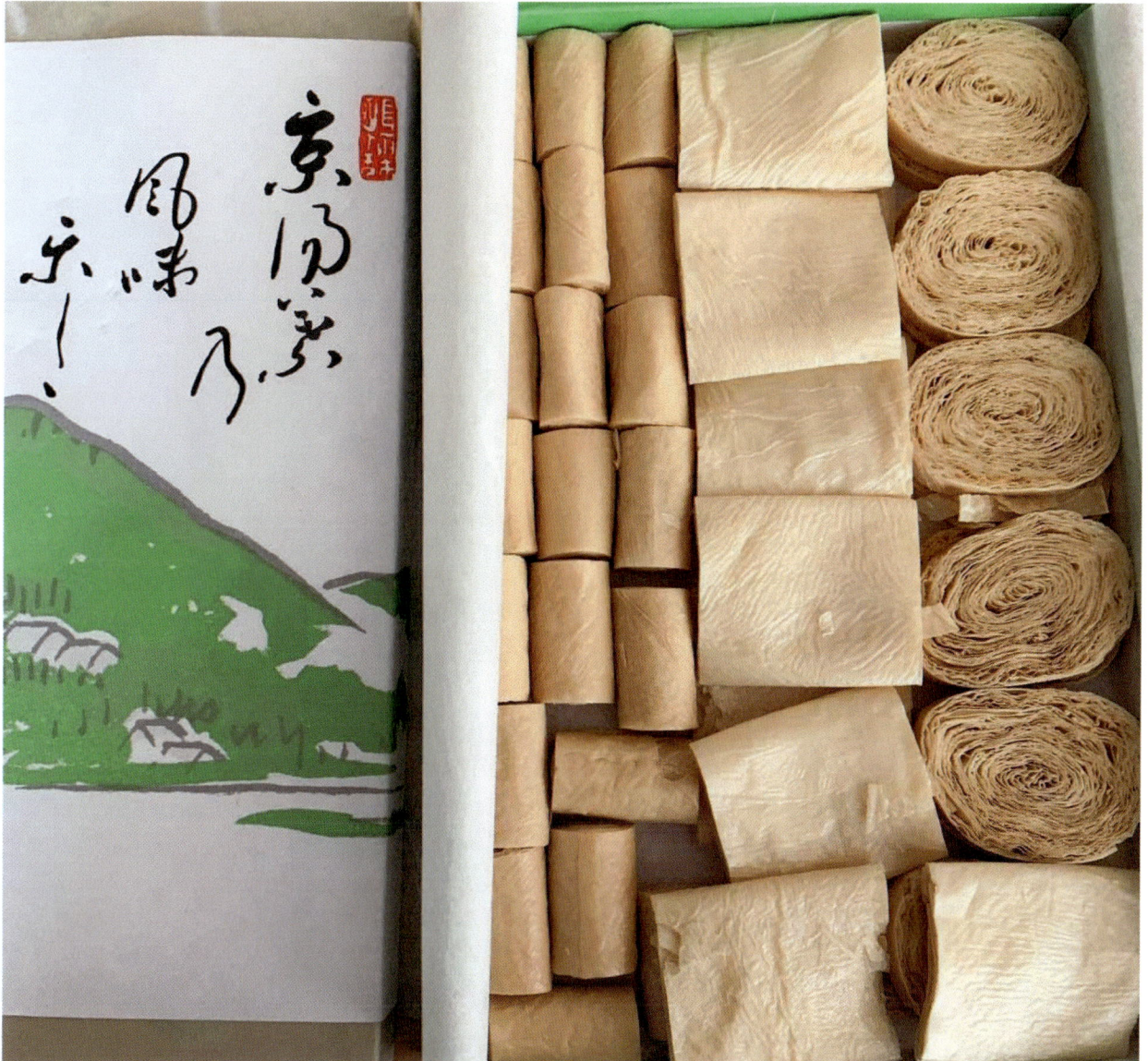

Dried yuba (soy milk skin)

Makes 2-3 servings

Ingredients

For the yuba

- 2 cups thick homemade soy milk, (double concentrated with 2 cups dried soy beans to 4 cups water)

For the an (あん sauce)

- 1 ½ cups dashi
- 1 Tbsp mirin
- 1 Tbsp sake
- 1 Tbsp soy sauce
- 1 Tbsp potato starch in 3 Tbsp water

Toppings - grated ginger, wasabi, green onion or shiso (perilla)

Directions

To make the yuba

1. If you have dried yuba, simply rehydrate the desired quantity in warm dashi for 15 minutes and set aside. Go straight to making the 'an' sauce.
2. If you're making the yuba from soy milk, pour the soy milk onto a wide pan and heat on medium low heat. After you notice the soy milk begin to simmer, it'll gradually form a skin after about 10 minutes.
3. You can gently touch the skin with a chopstick and see if it moves as one cohesive piece. If it doesn't, allow to cook a few more minutes until it has thickened. After it looks ready, detach the yuba from the sides of the pot and gently pick it up and transfer to a bowl.
4. In order to prevent the skins from sticking to each other, add unused soy milk to the bowl with yuba so the pieces are immersed in a soy milk bath.
5. Repeat steps 2 and 3, refilling the pan with fresh soy milk as needed, until all the soy milk is gone.

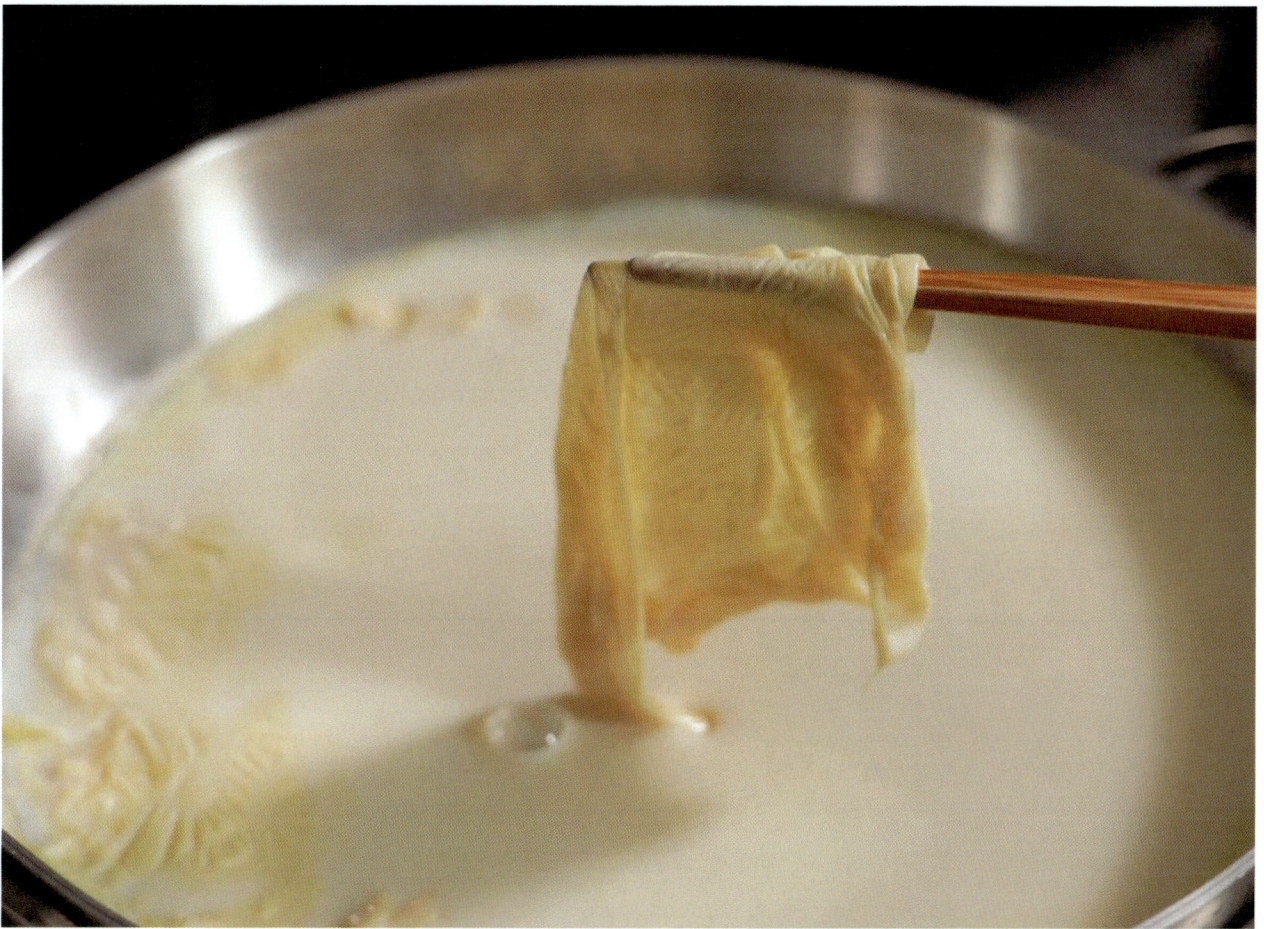

Making fresh yuba from homemade soy milk

To make the 'an' sauce

1. Combine the mirin, sake, soy sauce in a small pot and cook on medium heat until the alcohol has evaporated.
2. Get the potato starch slurry ready by stirring it to eliminate any clumps.
3. Gradually add the potato starch slurry into the dashi mixture stirring continuously to avoid clumping. Bring to a gentle boil and within a minute or so, the mixture should be noticeably thicker.
4. Once thickened, remove from heat and cover.

To serve, choose one of the following:

- Mix the yuba into the 'an' sauce and top a small bowl of rice with the mixture.
- Top the rice with the yuba first and then pour the 'an' sauce over it.

- **Tips:**

- In order to make yuba, you'll need fresh soy milk made with soy beans and water. If using store bought soy milk, double check the ingredients to ensure there is no flavoring or additives.
- Using two or more wide pans will help you make the yuba twice as fast if you're making the yuba from soy milk.
- When making the yuba, use medium low heat to avoid scorching the soy milk. Scorching will form a hard to clean crust on the bottom of your stainless or enameled pans. If this occurs, simply soak in water after finishing and use some Bar Keepers Friend to get any residual pieces off.
- You can also try using non-stick pans for easier clean up. I've experimented with using a pan on it's own and with a double boiler, and in my experience the soy milk sticks to my stainless pans either way.
- Try mixing in ginger, onion or shiso (perilla) leaves into the 'an' sauce for different combinations of flavors.

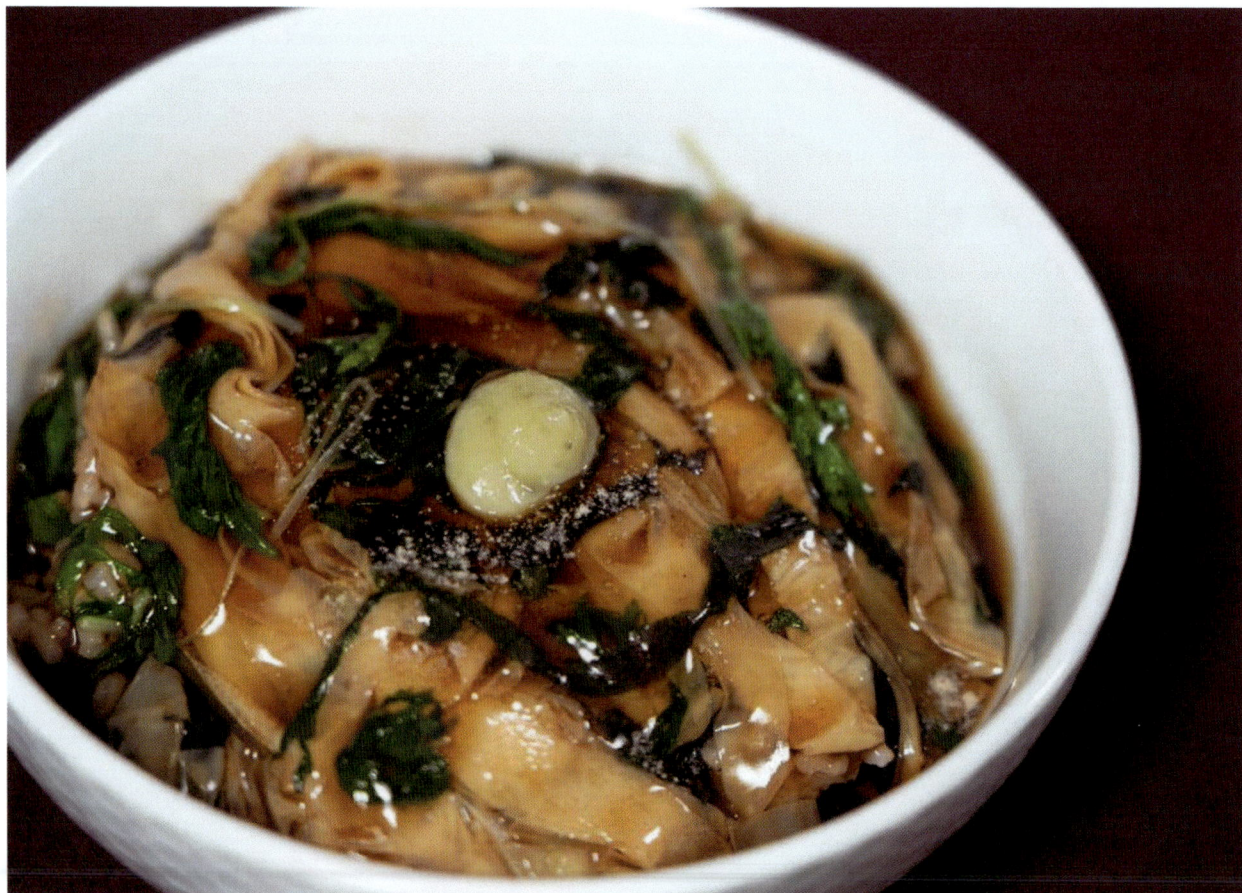

Yubadonburi with rehydrated yuba, red and green shiso, mizuna and wasabi

Gomoku takikomigohan
(Seasoned rice with 5 vegetables)
五目炊き込みご飯

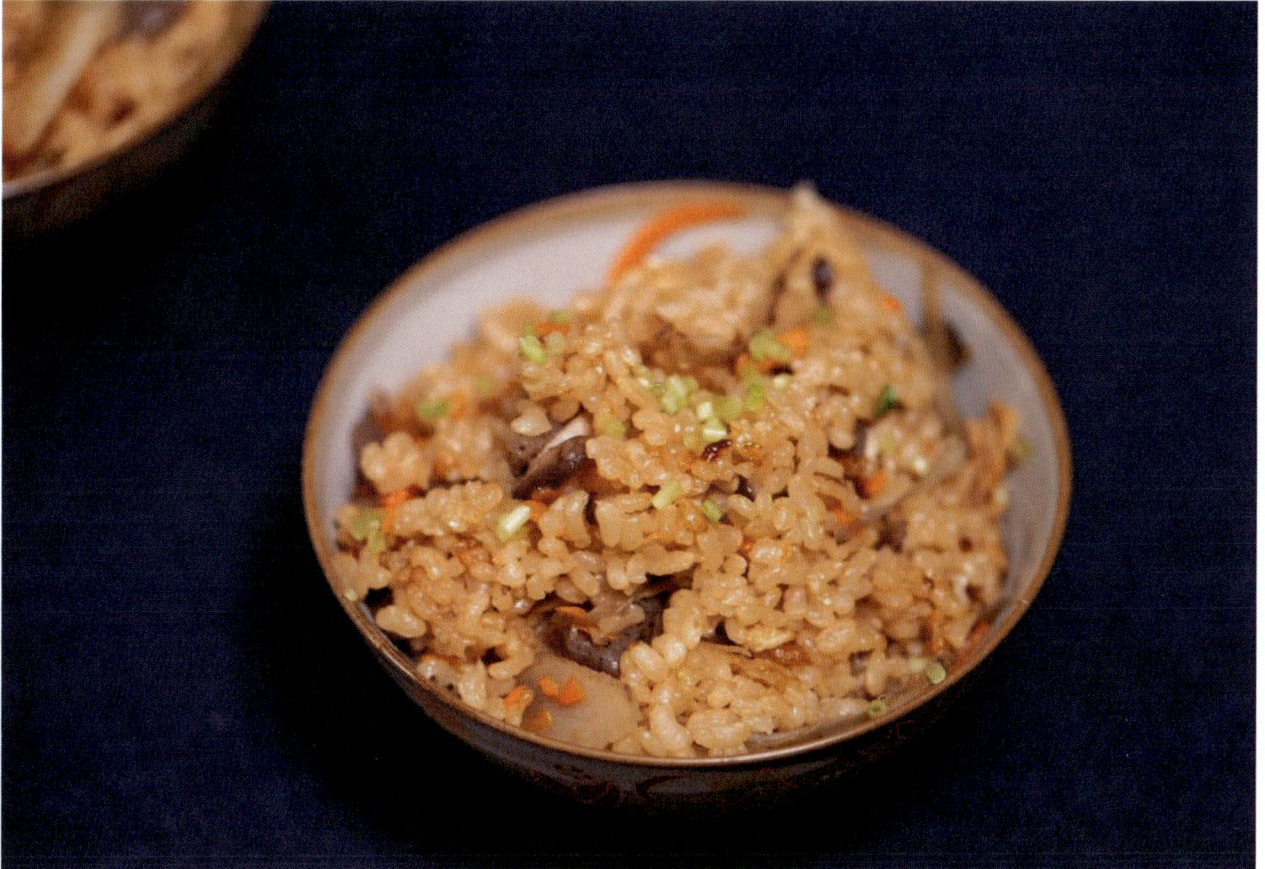

There may be a point in your Japanese cooking journey where plain white or brown rice may get old, if you're not there already.

If and when that happens, you can keep things interesting by adding tsukudani (佃煮 soy seasoned foods), otsukemono (お漬け物 pickles) or even furikake (ふりかけ rice seasoning). But even then, rice may still be boring.

So how do you fix it? Takikomigohan (炊き込みご飯 seasoned rice)!

Makes 5-6 servings

Ingredients

- 2 cups Japanese brown rice, (short grain)
- 1 cup fresh shiitake mushrooms, destemmed and thinly sliced
- 2 pieces aburaage, (fried tofu skins), cut into small strips
- ⅕ block konnyaku, parboiled for 2- 3 min and cut into strips
- 1 cup carrots, julienned
- 1 cup gobo, (burdock root) sasagaki *
- 1 Tbsp sake
- 1 Tbsp mirin
- 2 Tbsps soy sauce

Directions

1. Rinse the rice and add it to your rice cooker. Fill with water up to brown rice water level, then remove 5 tablespoons of water.
2. Add all of the vegetables to the rice cooker, but don't mix to ensure the rice cooks evenly.
3. Add in the seasonings and cook.
4. Once the rice is done, gently fold the vegetables into the rice to evenly distribute.
5. Serve warm.

Tips:

- Check which cup measurements your rice cooker uses to avoid mushy rice. Japanese cups are different from American cups, so make sure to use the measuring cup that came with your rice cooker. Alternatively, if using an American cup measure, follow the liquid to rice ratio on the pack.
- *For gobo, refer to the okara misoshiru tips on page 35.
- Instead of water, you can also use dashi for additional flavor. I alternate between the two depending on my mood or if I have dashi ready to use.
- A good substitute for konnyaku strips are shirataki noodles (miracle noodles). Both are made from the same ingredients and provide a nice chewy texture which complements the other vegetables and textures in this dish. If substituting, use ¼ cup of shirataki noodles in place of the konnyaku. I recommend parboiling the noodles as you would the konnyaku to improve flavor and texture.

Shiokouji (Salted fermented rice)

塩麹

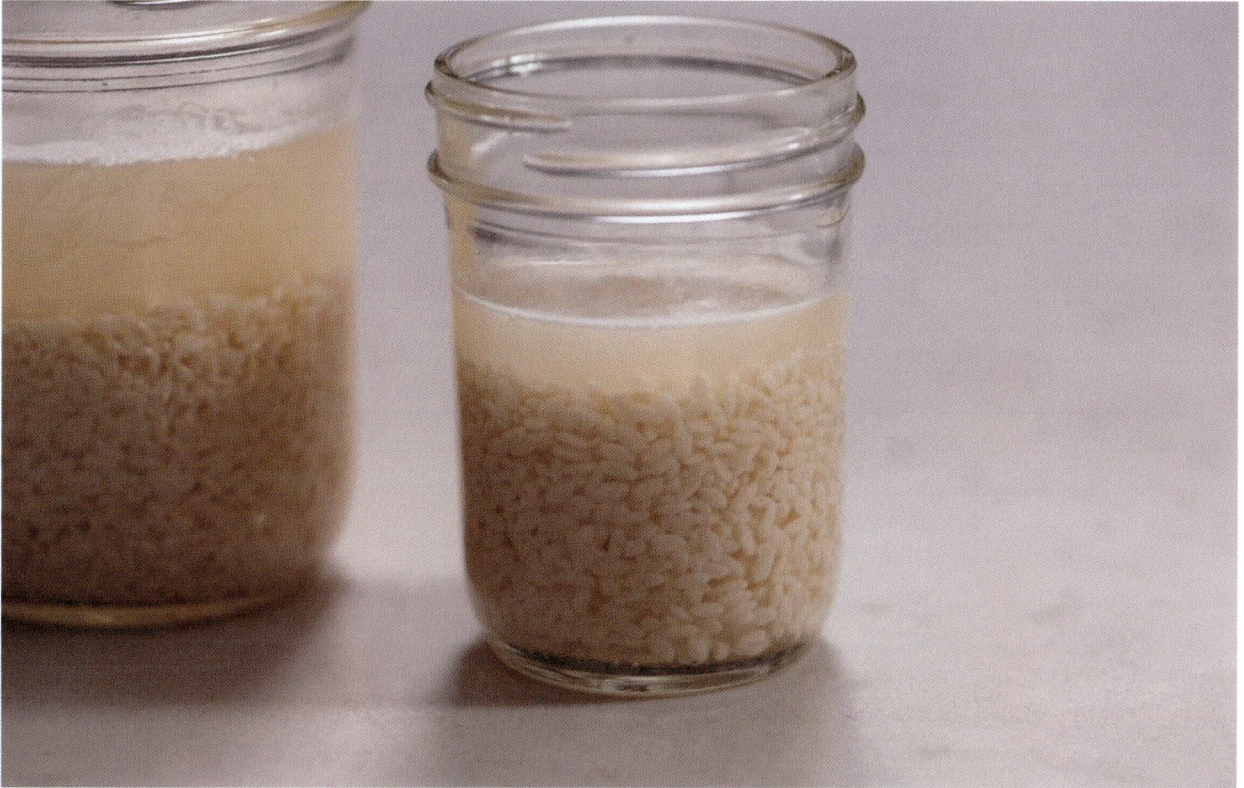

Shiokouji is made with komekouji (米麹 rice inoculated with aspergillus oryzae mold). The komekouji is mixed with water and salt and allowed to ferment at room temperature for at least 5 -10 days. The result is a thick, salty, slightly sweet, slightly funky, multipurpose condiment that can enhance the flavor and texture of your food.

Shiokouji works its magic in several ways. It gently dehydrates foods at the surface and also breaks down proteins into their building blocks (amino acids). The breakdown of proteins helps to improve texture and the freed amino acids naturally enhance the flavor of food (with umami)!

Use shiokouji just like salt but when you want additional flavor and complexity.

As you may know, shiokouji is just one of many kouji products. Kouji (麹 aspergillus) is the same mold that's used to make sake, as well as, soy sauce and miso! While you can make each of those yourself, they do require a good amount of time before you can enjoy them.

On the other hand, simple kouji products that can be made quickly include: shouyu kouji (醤油麹 soy sauce kouji) and amakouji (甘麹 sweet kouji). Both of these have unique complex flavors which can be used as substitutes for soy sauce or sugar respectively.

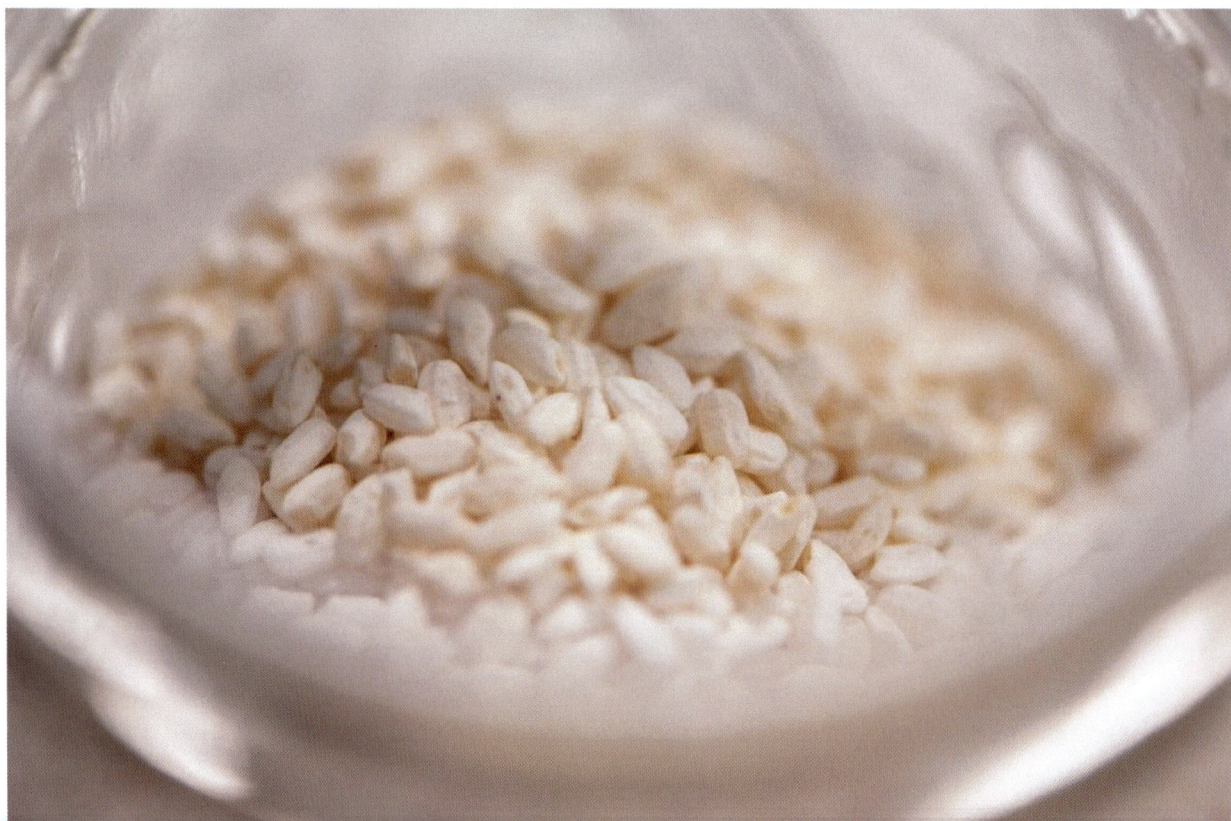

Komekouji

Kyabetsu takikomigohan
(Seasoned rice with red cabbage)
キャベツ炊き込みご飯

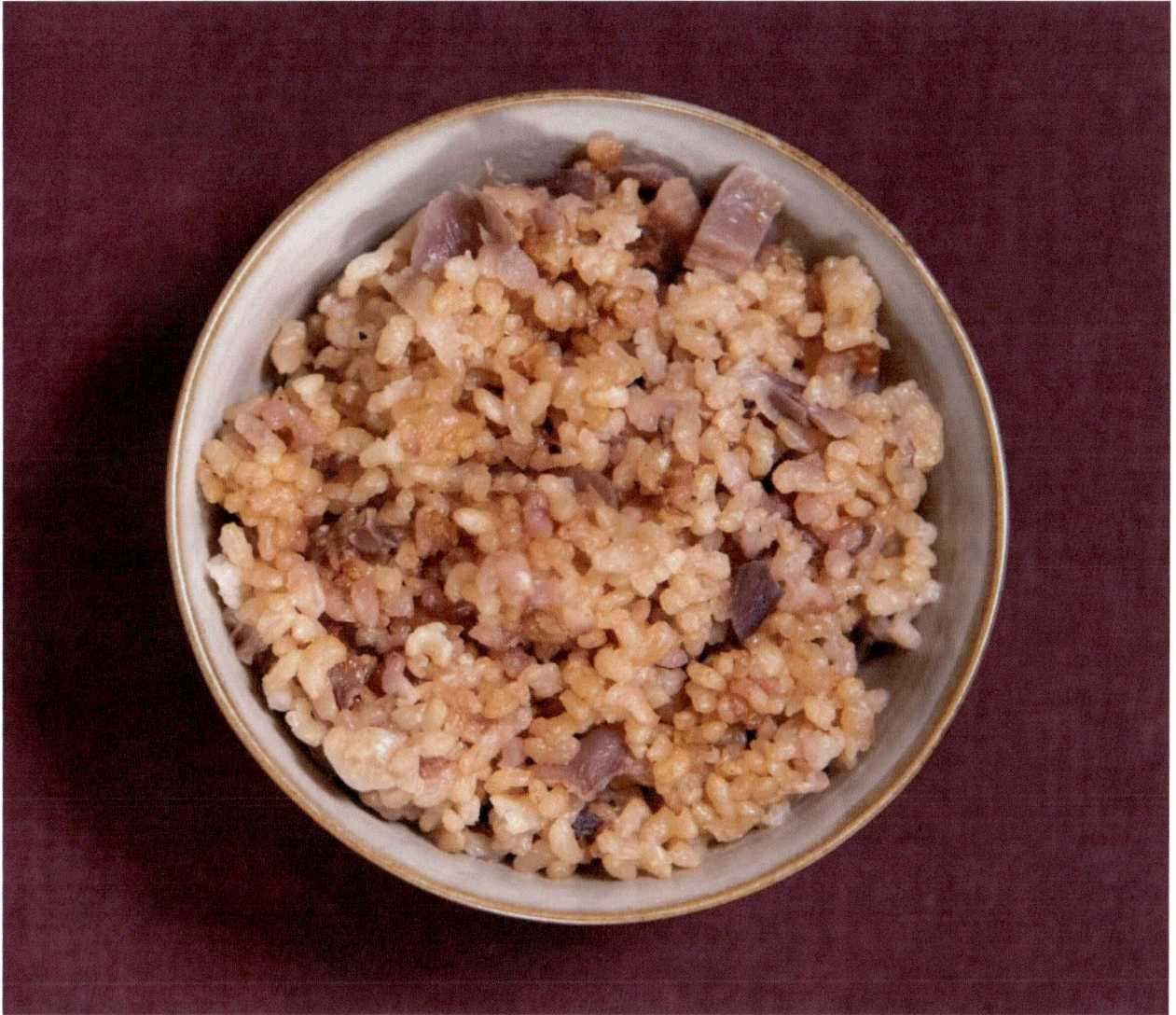

What makes this version of takikomigohan special is that it's full of flavor thanks to the miso, dashi, and shiokouji. It's something I usually double for leftovers for days I don't feel like cooking and it freezes well too!

Makes 5-6 servings

Ingredients

- 2 cups Japanese brown rice, (short grain)
- 2 Tbsps light soy sauce, (usukuchi shouyu)
- 2 cups konbu dashi or konbu shiitake dashi *(enough to fill to the 2-cup line of rice cooker or follow pack directions for water:rice ratio)*
- 1-2 Tbsps ginger, cut into thin matchsticks
- ¼ head red cabbage, finely chopped or thinly sliced
- ¼ onion, chopped
- 1 Tbsp sesame oil
- 1 tsp red miso paste
- 1 tsp shiokouji or ⅓ tsp salt
- Freshly cracked black pepper

Directions

1. Using a saucepan on medium heat, add sesame oil and cook the cabbage, ginger, and onion.
2. After 3 minutes, add in the miso paste, shiokouji, freshly cracked black pepper, and mix thoroughly.
3. Cook on medium low heat for 5- 7 minutes until the vegetables have softened.
4. Rinse the brown rice, drain thoroughly, and add to your rice cooker.
6. Add the light soy sauce and enough dashi to the 2 cup water line, then add the vegetables and cook the rice.
7. Once the rice is done, gently fold the vegetables into the rice to evenly distribute.
5. Serve warm.

Tips:

- In my rice cooker, I always slightly under fill the water level, so that the water is just under the hatch mark. This always results in a firmer drier rice, which is the way I like it. If you haven't already, test different water levels to see the effect it has on texture and find out what you like best.
- Make this rice two ways: takikomigohan where you cook everything in the rice cooker or as mazegohan (混ぜご飯 mixed rice), where you cook the rice first then add the cooked vegetables to the cooked rice by mixing it in. Try both and see if you prefer one over the other.

Shiokouji kyuri
(Cucumber with shiokouji)
塩麹キュウリ

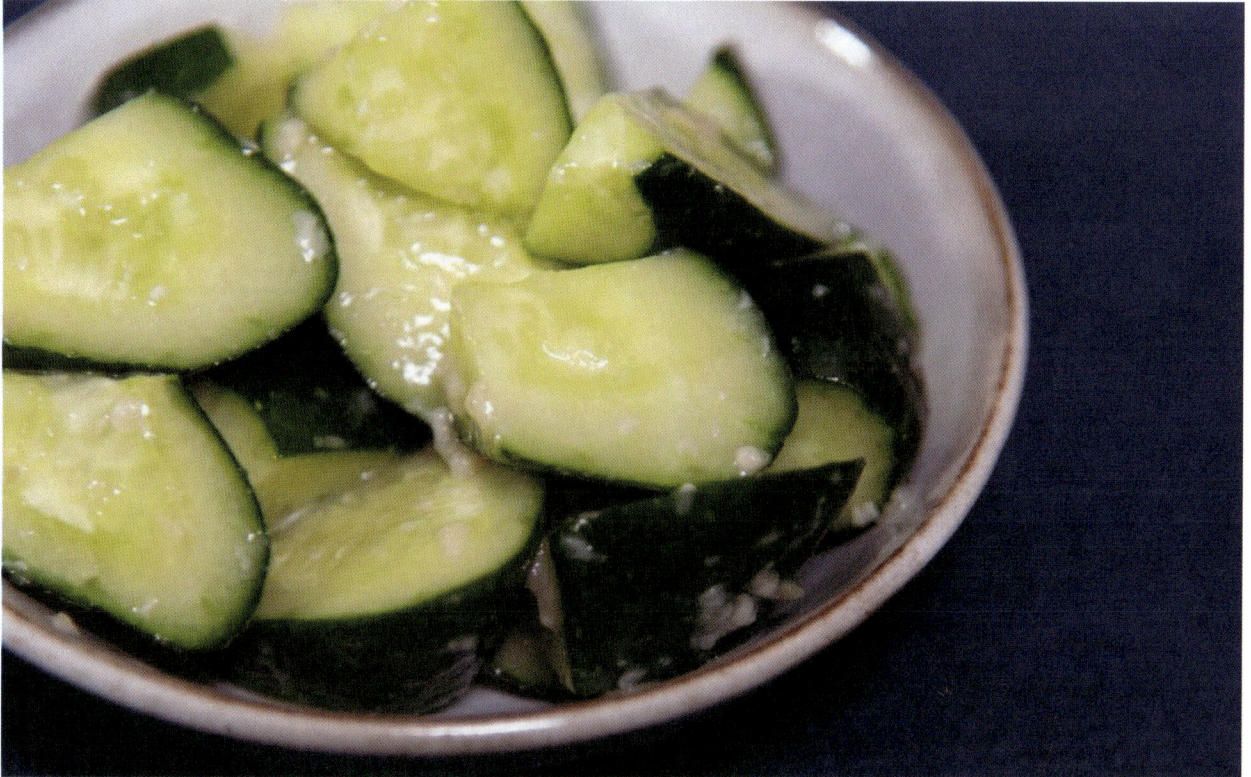

Cucumbers are a refreshing way to add some vegetables to your meal and especially so with a somewhat spicy invisible ingredient...wasabi!

You'd never know it was there just by looking at it. Wanna surprise someone? ;) But if you got close enough to give it a whiff, you might pick up on it, and you'd definitely know as you're eating it.

If you love wasabi you'll love these cucumbers. And if you don't, a good replacement would be something like grated ginger.

Makes 4-6 servings

Ingredients

- 2 Japanese cucumbers (~3 cups), rangiri*
- 1 Tbsp shiokouji
- 1 tsp wasabi paste

Directions

1. Mix the cucumber with shiokouji and wasabi so each piece is evenly coated.
2. Allow to rest in the refrigerator for at least 15 minutes.
3. Serve chilled.

Tips:

- *Rangiri, refer to kenchinjiru recipe tips on page 39.
- Shiokouji is salty so it will draw out moisture from the food you're using it on. With vegetables especially - if you don't plan on eating it right away, don't mix together until about 15-30 minutes prior to eating. If you have leftovers, you'll notice that water will get drawn out and dilute your seasoning the next day.
- Think of these cucumbers as pickles; you only need to eat a little bit in between bites of the other parts of your meal!
- Try to use real wasabi. It tastes way better than any tube or powder form and when grated, fresh wasabi offers a nice refreshing and awakening sensation unlike any other ingredient! For the longest time I disliked wasabi because most often often than not it's made with horseradish, which I really dislike. But once I had the real thing, fresh real wasabi soon became one of my favorite ingredients.
- Real wasabi can be found online. Visit alldayieat.com/go/bookresources for more info.

Shiokouji moyashi
(Bean sprouts with shiokouji)
もやし塩麹

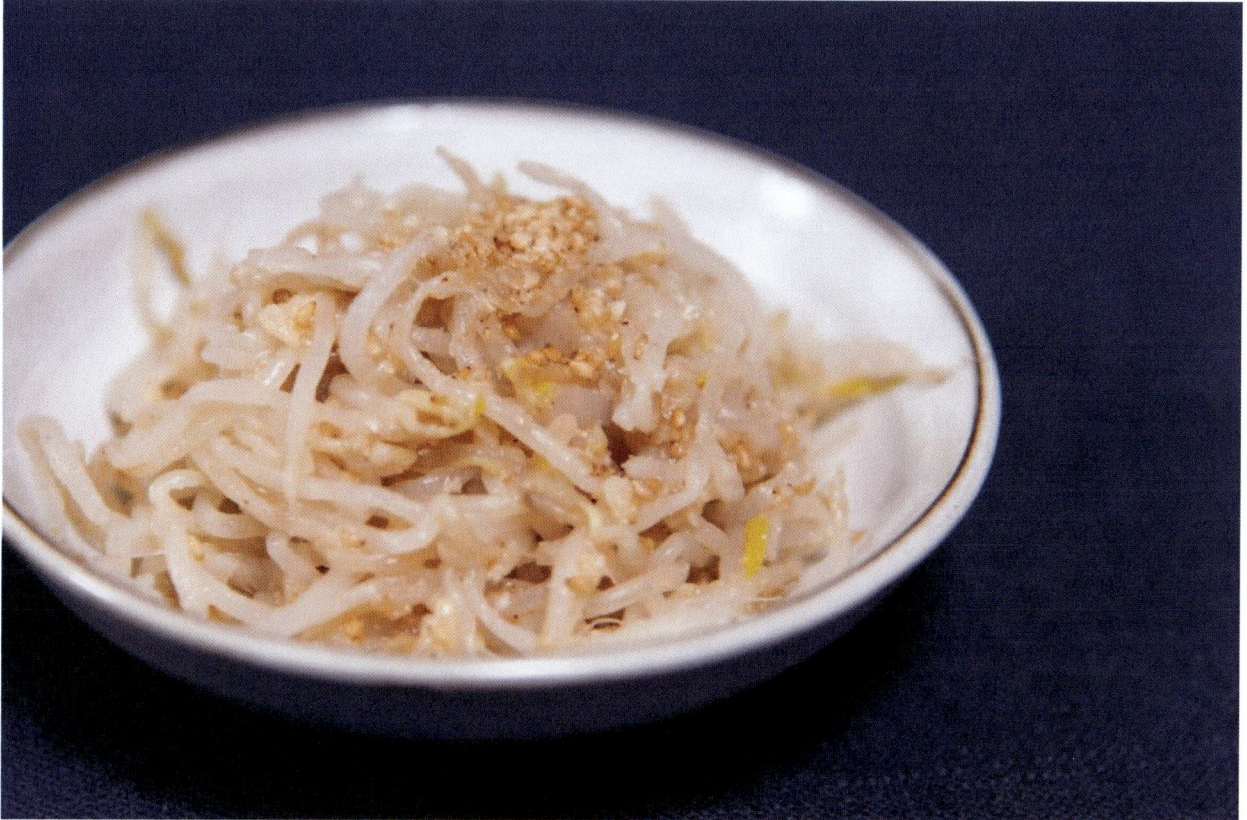

Bean sprouts are a delicious way to enjoy shiokouji. The mild flavor of the bean sprouts are accentuated by both the sesame and the funky, slightly complex flavor of shiokouji!

This is similar to gomaae (ごま和え sesame soy-dressed vegetables) but without the soy sauce.

Like gomaae, this makes for a refreshing and tasty side dish that's simple to make.

Makes 4 servings

Ingredients

- 1 bag mung bean sprouts (9 oz.)
- 3 Tbsps white sesame seeds, toasted and ground
- 2 Tbsps shiokouji
- Optional - dash of sesame oil

Directions

1. Prepare a large pot of lightly salted water and bring to a boil.
2. Blanch the bean sprouts for 30-45 seconds so they have a little bite left.
3. Drain immediately, and chill with cold water and or an ice bath if you prefer cold bean sprouts. Once chilled, squeeze out the excess water.
4. Prepare the dressing by mixing 2 tablespoons of ground sesame seeds, the shiokouji, and sesame oil if using.
5. Mix the dressing with the bean sprouts
6. Allow to rest for 15 minutes for the shiokouji to work it's magic!
7. Top with the remaining tablespoon of ground sesame seeds and serve at room temperature or chilled.

Tips:

- Depending on how much water remains in the bean sprouts, the shiokouji may make this salty. Different brands of shiokouji have different levels of salt as would making your own homemade shiokouji. When using shiokouji for the first time, start with than 1 - 1 ½ tablespoons to be a little more conservative. As with salt, you can always add more but you can't take it out.
- As with gomaae, you can use black sesame seeds for a different flavor or even a mixture of the two to change things up.
- For a tasty twist, add in ¼ cup nira (garlic chives) or a couple of stalks of green onion. Briefly blanch both and then cut into small strips the size of the bean sprouts. This will add a mild garlic or onion flavor to the dish.

Namasu (Pickled carrot and daikon)
塩麹なます

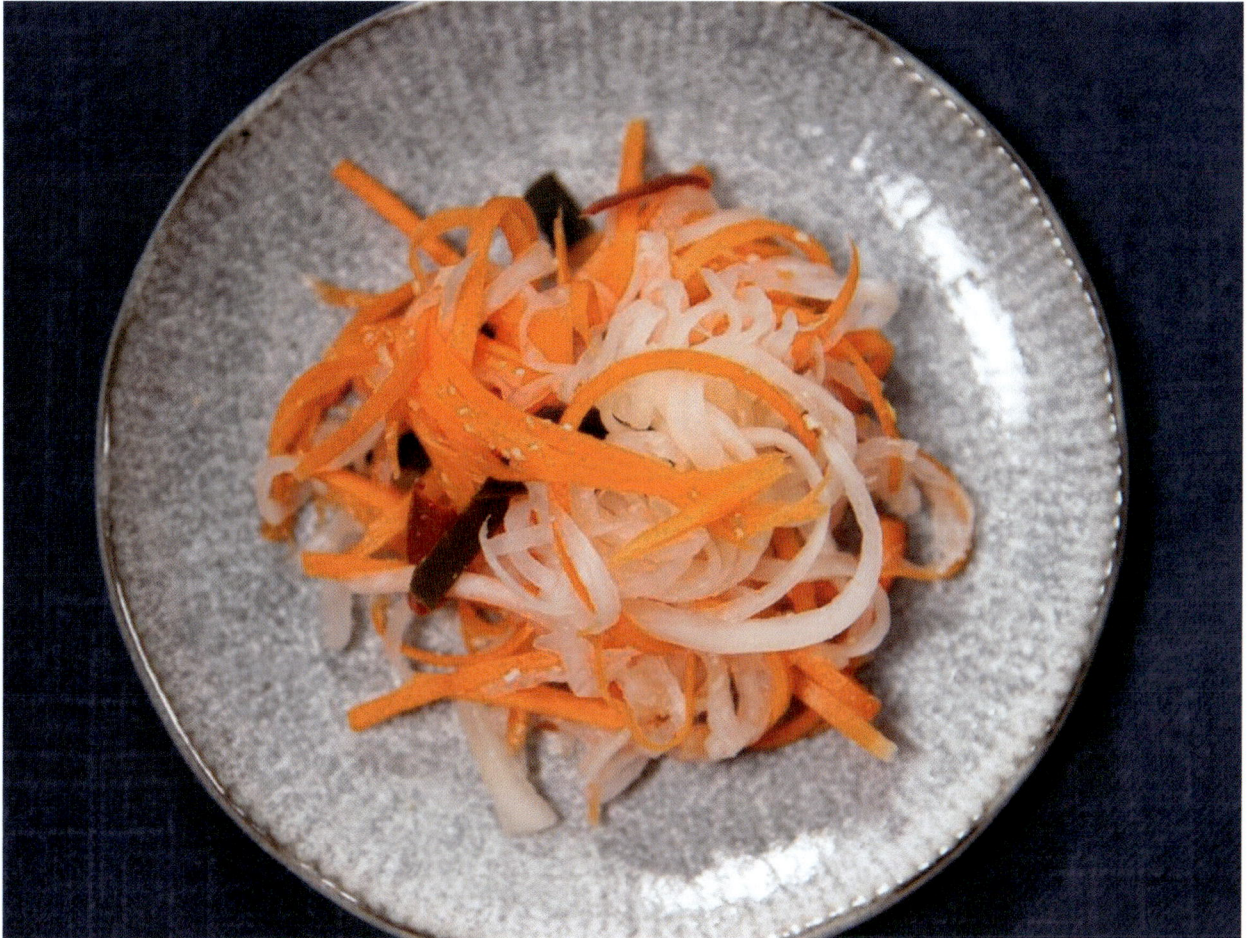

Namasu literally translated means 'raw vinegar.' The 'raw' is the vegetable and the vinegar is what's used to season the vegetables.

The combination of daikon radish and carrot is a delicious mixture of savory and sweet and both are made that much better thanks to the help of konbu dashi and shiokouji!!

Makes 8 servings

Ingredients

- 3-4 cups daikon radish, peeled and julienned
- 2 cups carrots, peeled and julienned
- 2 Tbsps shiokouji
- 2 x 3 in. piece dashigarakonbu, (leftover konbu from making dashi) chopped into small matchsticks

For the seasoning

- 2 tsps shiokouji
- 3 Tbsps rice vinegar
- 2 tsps white sugar
- 3 Tbsps konbu dashi
- 1 red chili with seeds, chopped, or 1 tsp red pepper

Directions

1. Combine the daikon and carrots with shiokouji in a plastic bag or glass bowl. Mix thoroughly so all pieces are evenly coated and allow to rest at least 20 minutes.
2. Prepare your seasoning by combining all the seasoning ingredients into a jar and set aside.
3. Once the daikon/carrot mixture has rested for 20 minutes, drain. Squeeze gently to extract most of the water.
4. Combine the seasoning with daikon/carrot mixture, the dashigarakonbu, and red chili.
5. Reuse the same bag or a glass bowl and marinate in the refrigerator for at least 2 hours before serving.

Tips:

- This is one of those okazu (**おかず** side dish) that's meant to be eaten in small quantities - about ¼ cup or less per person. It goes well with many different foods, providing some pleasant acidity to cleanse and refresh your palate.
- Depending on the season, daikon radish may be more 'spicy' or bitter in the summer and milder or sweeter in the winter. If you find that you're sensitive to it, you can let the namasu rest a few days and you'll notice the spicy/bitterness will have mellowed out.
- You can vary the ratio of daikon to carrots- I personally like a 2:1 ratio, but try to keep the volume the same so you don't end up with a seasoning too strong or too diluted.
- Since it's pickled, it keeps well for up to 7 days, by which date we usually eat it all so I can't really say if it'll last longer than that!

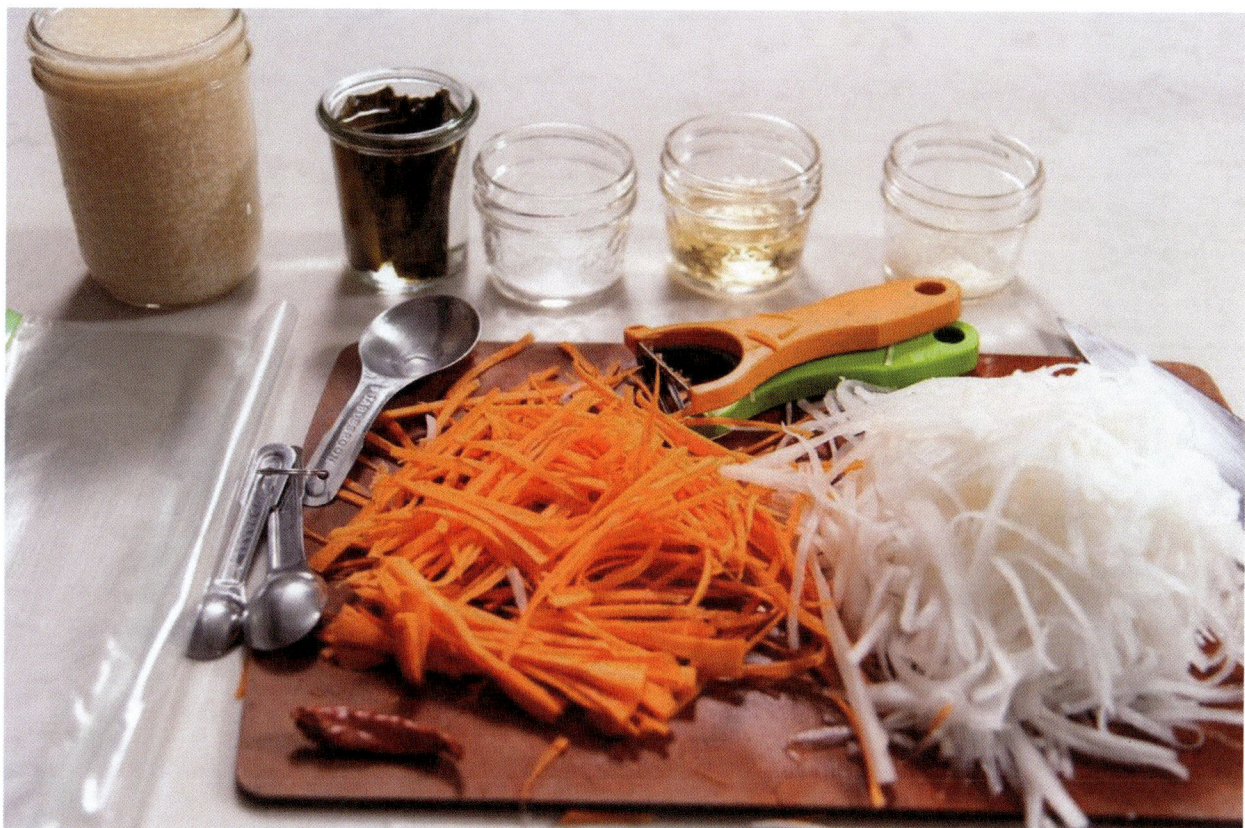

Namasu ingredients

Kabocha supu (Kabocha squash soup)
南瓜スープ

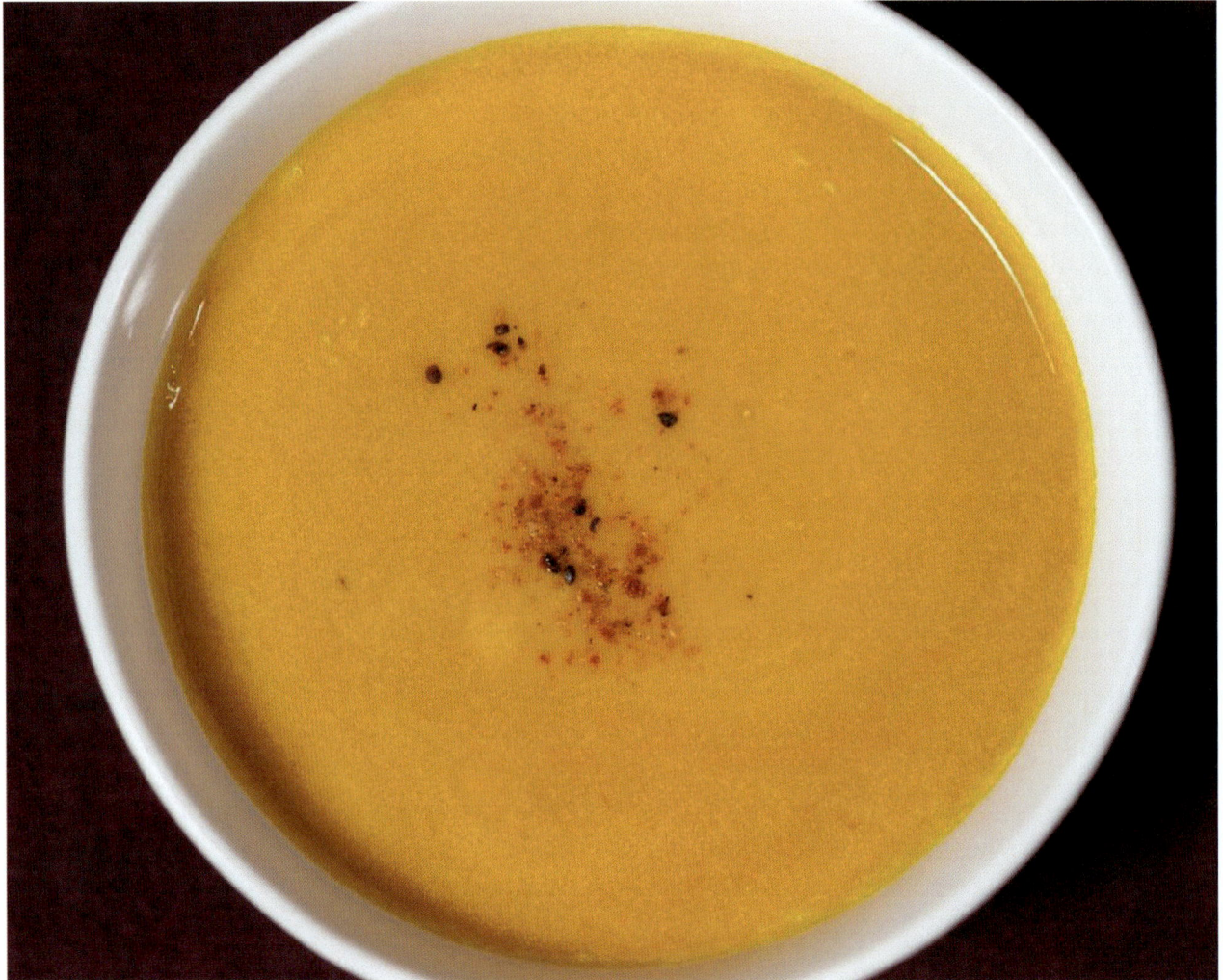

Kabocha is one of my favorite vegetables.

How about you?

One of the reasons for me is that there are so many different ways to enjoy it. Ranging from savory to sweet, some of my favorites would have to be in a Japanese dessert like purin (プリン pudding) or in a soup, just like this one!

Makes 5-6 servings

Ingredients

- 1 cup caramelized onion
- 1 medium kabocha (~ 2 lbs), deseeded, top and bottom stem removed*
- 4 cups soy milk
- 2 Tbsps sake
- 2 Tbsps shiokouji

Toppings- chopped green onions, chives, toasted pepitas, black and/or white pepper, shichimi pepper.

Directions

1. Using a large pot, add the caramelized onion, kabocha, soy milk, sake and shiokouji.
2. Bring to a gentle simmer and cook partially covered for about 15 minutes. Check the kabocha pieces for doneness by piercing with a chopstick (it should go through with little resistance).
3. Once the kabocha is cooked, use an immersion blender or regular blender to puree. *Be extra careful with this hot mixture!*
4. Serve with desired toppings as a side or with a bowl of brown rice for a light meal!

Tips:

- Caramelizing the onion adds depth and complexity to the soup. If you aren't keen on taking the time to make it, consider waiting until you have the time and make an extra large batch! That way you can use them in other recipes too!
- *Soften the kabocha before cooking by microwaving on high power at least 5 minutes. This also helps to partially cook the flesh, reducing cooking time.
- A few things to consider when working with kabocha-
  - To get a deep orange color of soup, remove the skin of the kabocha. Yes, it's got fiber and nutrition, but the skin makes the color of your soup more of a pale orange, while it's not unappetizing (at least to me), it may not be as appealing to look at as when it's made without. Beauty is in the eye of the beholder, so you decide!

  - You can save the kabocha skin for a different soup or toss them in after you've taken your pictures ;)

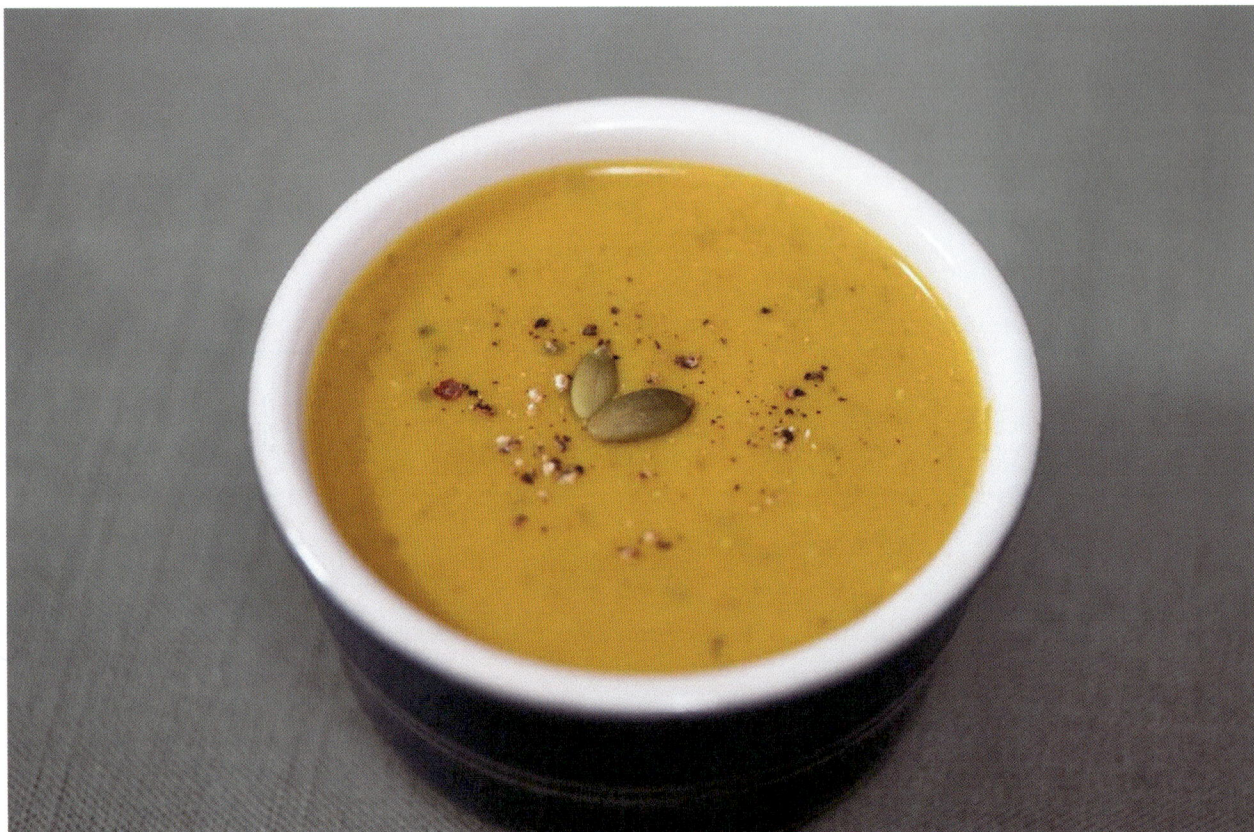

Kabocha soup with skin

Otsukemono (Japanese pickles)

お漬け物

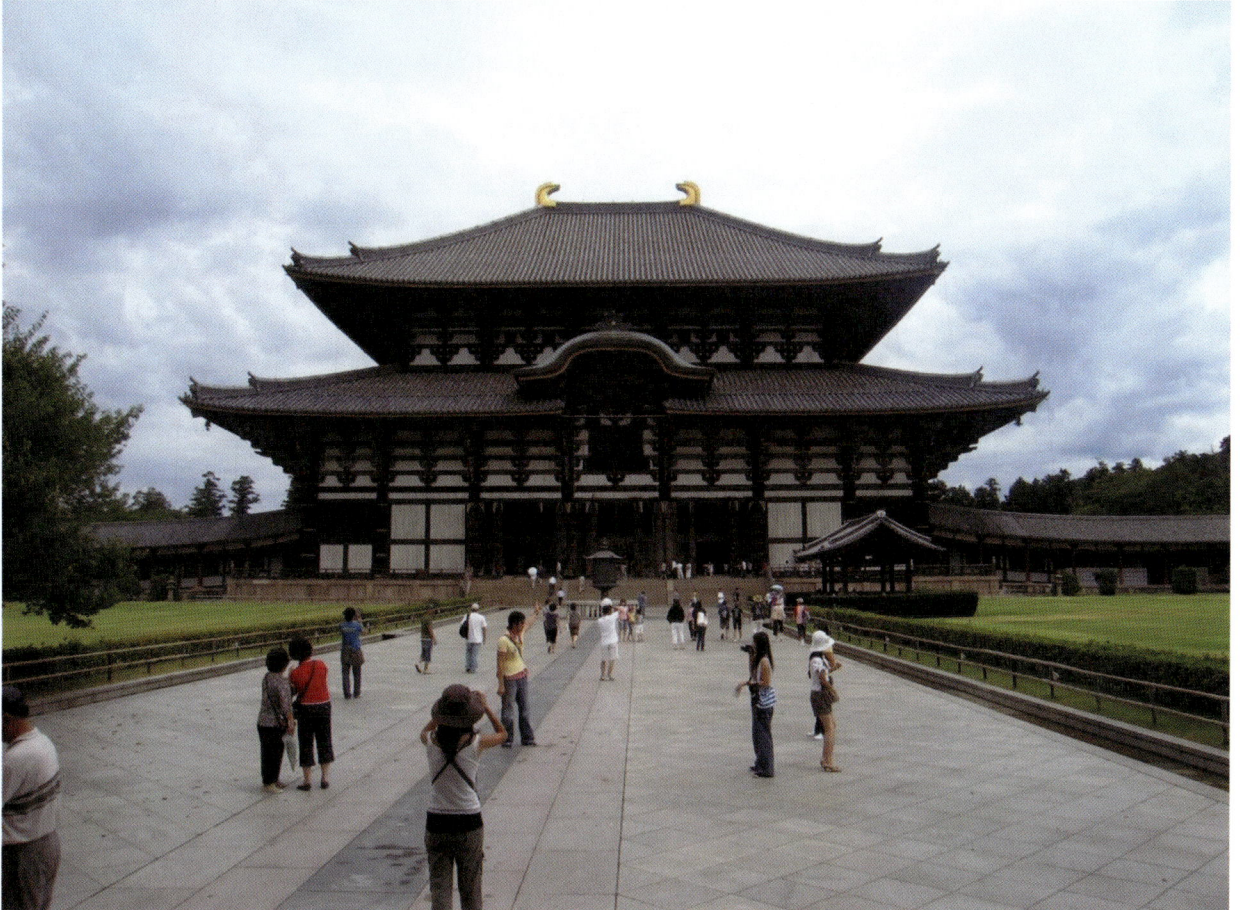

Todaiji, Nara, Japan

Curious to know what Nara and otsukemono have in common? The Nara region is famous not only for its temples, but also for its own distinctive type of Japanese pickles narazuke (奈良漬 Nara style pickles).

As you may know, pickles are a fundamental part of a traditional Japanese meal. If you're in a restaurant having a teishoku (定食 set meal) or a traditional meal with rice and soup, chances are you'll be served at least one type of otsukemono.

Otsukemono is a good way to not only to add some unique flavors and textures to your meal, but also get some more vegetables into your diet. And if you grow your own, it's a great way to preserve them!

In this next section, we'll make a few of my favorites using easy to find ingredients. It may help to get an otsukemono press, but like any tool, it's not necessary, it just makes the job easier.

As well as tasting amazingly fresh and light, the best part about making your own otsukemono is that it won't be too salty or have any of the artificial colors or additives like MSG often used in store-bought varieties.

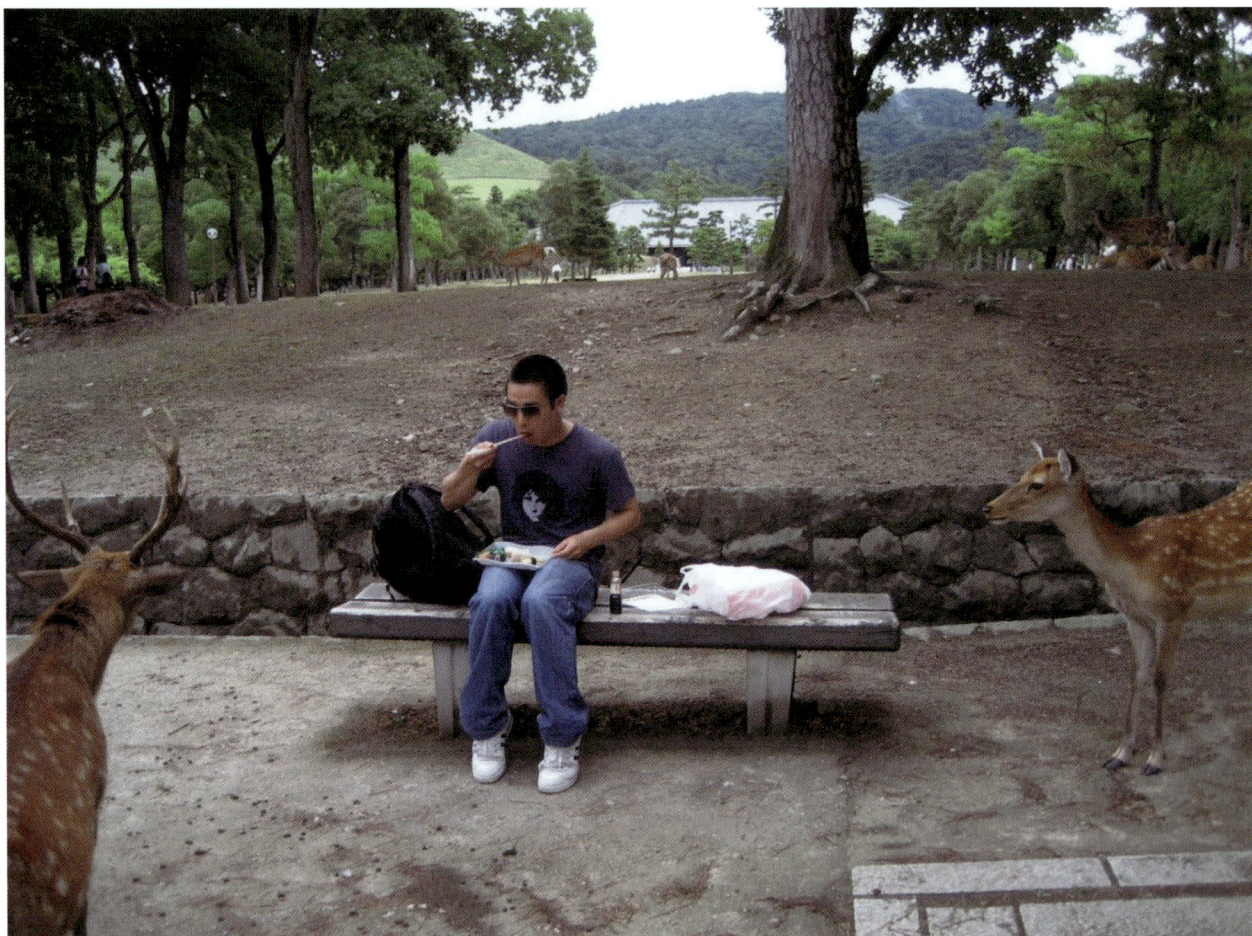

Protecting my lunch from the deer Nara, Japan

Hakusai otsukemono (Pickled napa cabbage)
白菜お漬物

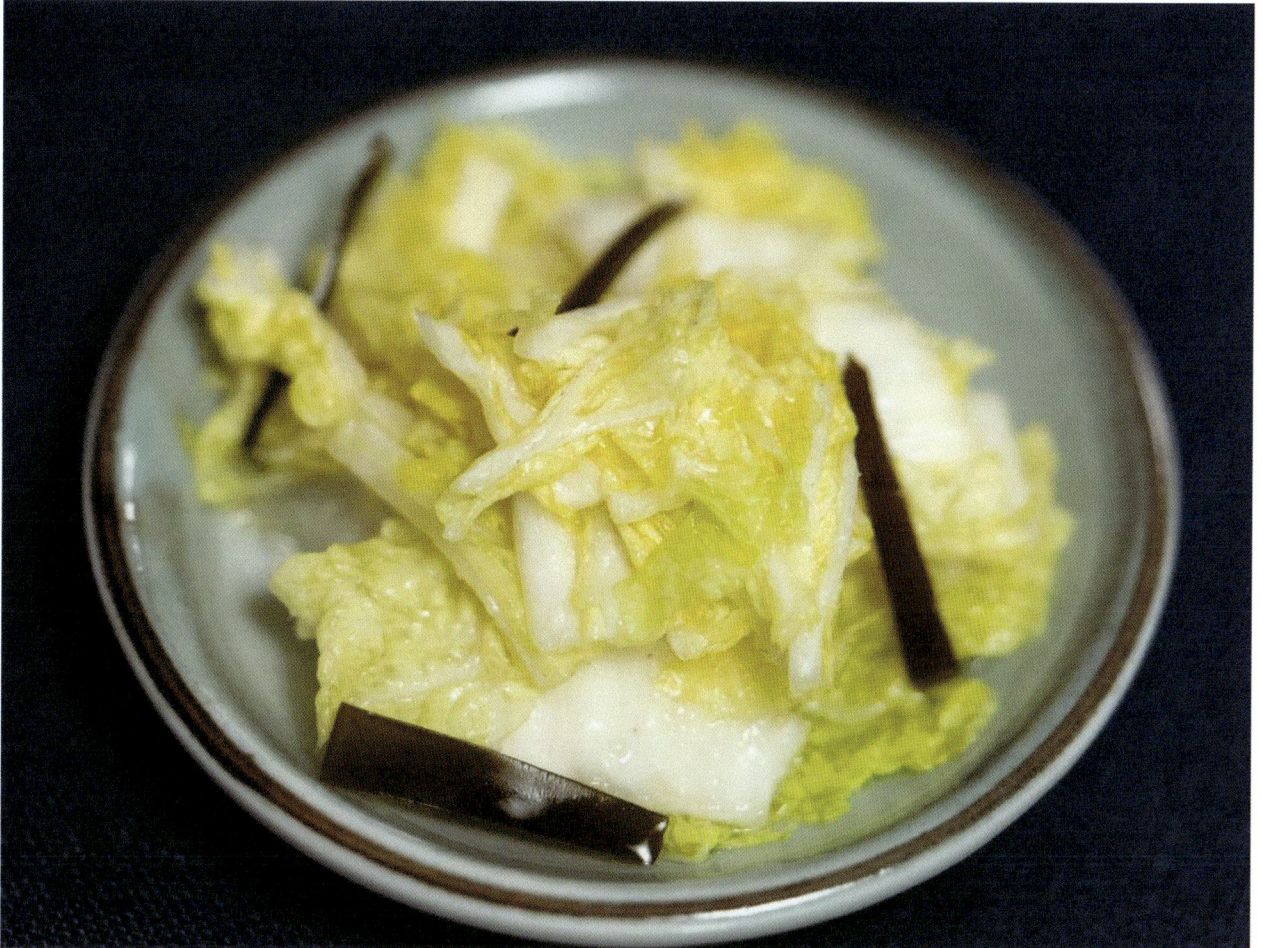

This pickled napa cabbage is a very common and simple Japanese pickle. It's tasty and light, and goes with almost any type of meal.

If you like a little bit of spice, consider adding a red chili pepper or red pepper flakes.

Makes 1 pint

Ingredients

- 1 lb. napa cabbage, root removed and cut into 1 in. pieces
- 9 g salt (2% total weight of cabbage)
- 4 g konbu (1% total weight of cabbage)
- Optional - red pepper flakes

Directions

1. Lightly toast the konbu over a small open flame to soften and cut into thin strips.
2. In the otsukemono press, mix the salt with the cabbage and konbu strips (and red pepper if using).
3. Place the lid on and screw down to apply pressure to the vegetables.
4. Allow to rest at least 3-4 hours.
5. When the liquid pools or comes out, make sure to drain.
6. Serve or use within 4-5 days.

Tips:

- Gently warming the konbu over an open flame helps to soften it before cutting. If you don't do this, the konbu will shatter into small pieces when cutting and make a mess.
- Use an otsukemono press if you can. It will make cleanup and the process a lot easier. If you don't have use two large bowls with a weight on top.
- Back in the day, what my grandmothers did in Japan, and even when they moved to the U.S., was to use clean large rocks (this was before the plastic presses like the one below were widely available).
- Serve with some lemon juice if you'd like a little citrus flavor.

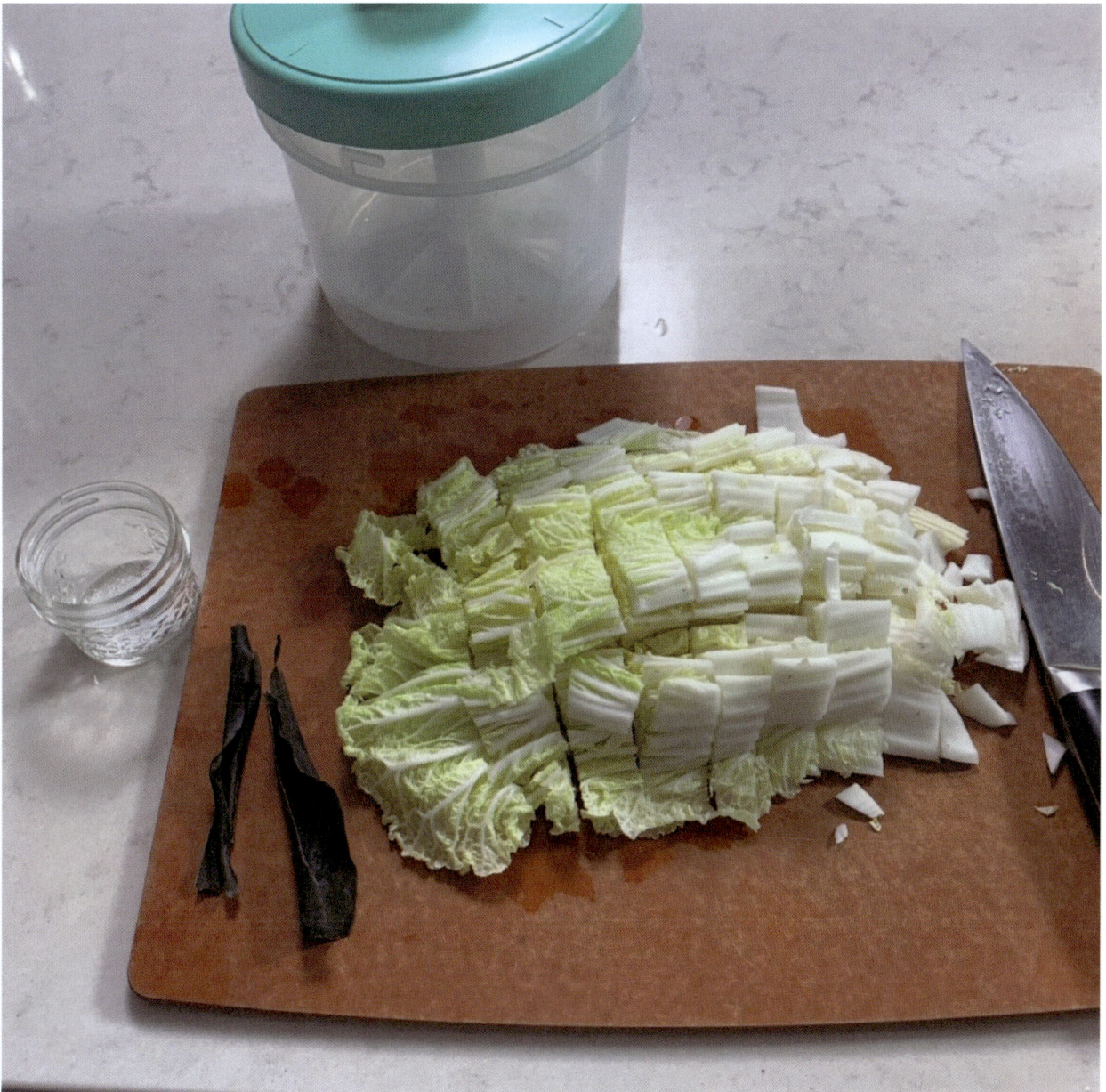

Ingredients for napa cabbage otsukemono

Daikon otsukemono (Pickled daikon)

大根お漬物物

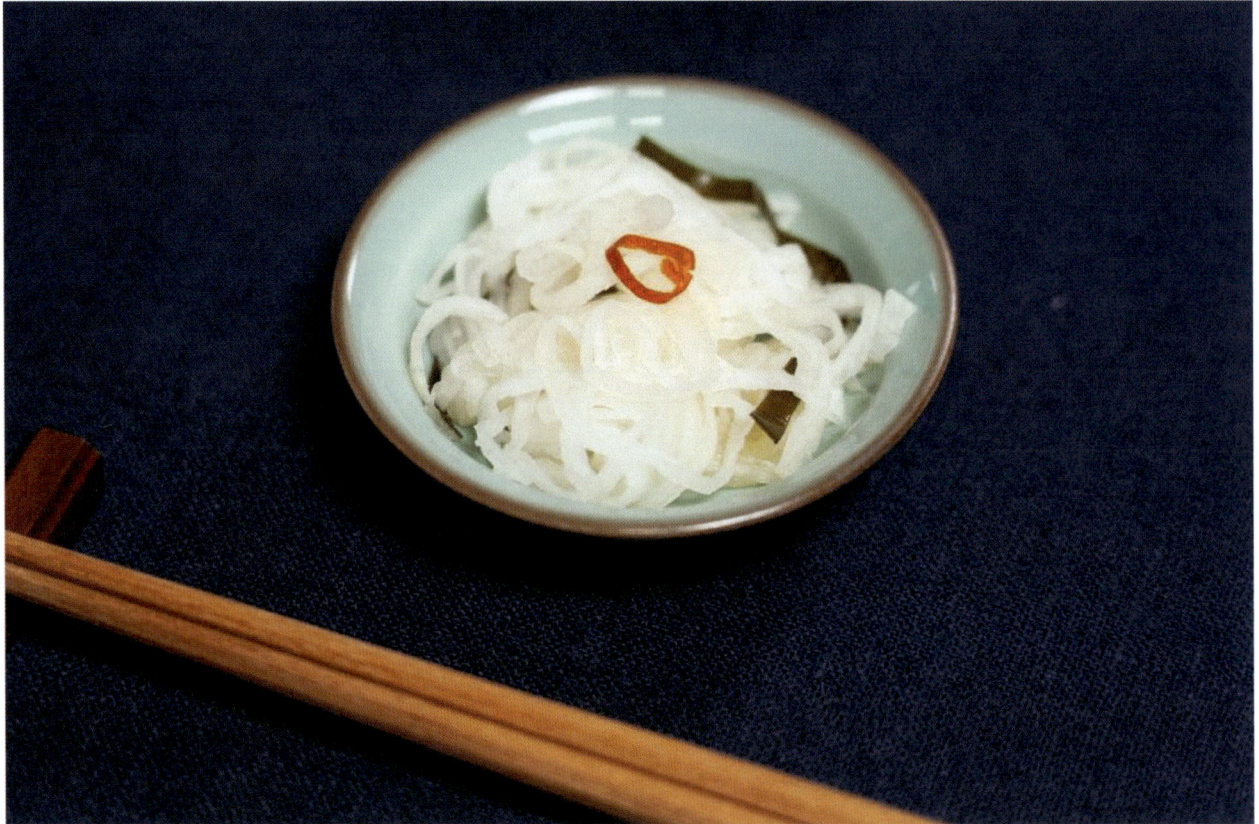

Here's another way for you to enjoy daikon radish.

Just like the napa cabbage recipe on the previous page, this one only requires a few ingredients and can be served with many different types of dishes.

Because daikon has a light and refreshing flavor, it's very suitable for pickling.

Makes 1 pint

Ingredients

- 1 lb. daikon radish, peeled and julienned
- 9 g salt (2% total weight of daikon)
- 4 g konbu (1% total weight of daikon)
- Optional: 1 dried red chili, deseeded and sliced thinly

Directions

1. Lightly toast the konbu over a small open flame to soften and cut into thin strips.
2. In an otsukemono press, mix the salt with the daikon, konbu strips, and red chili if using.
3. Place the lid on and screw down to apply pressure to the vegetables.
4. Allow to pickle at least 4-6 hours.
5. When the liquid pools or comes out, make sure to drain.
6. Serve and use within 4-5 days.

Tips:

- If you're lucky and get the radish tops, you can include those too and that'll give you a nice green color to contrast with the chili. To use the radish tops:
  - Discard any of the tough/fibrous leaves.
  - Blanch them for 1 minute in salted water and then shock them in an ice bath to stop the cooking.
  - Once cooled drain and dry thoroughly, and cut into very fine pieces
  - Mix in with the julienned daikon before pressing.
- Cut the daikon into different shapes to vary the presentation style. You can experiment with thin matchsticks, thin round slices or thin half-circles to change things up. The important thing to remember is to cut the daikon thinly. This will help it to season evenly and for extra water to be drawn out when pressed.

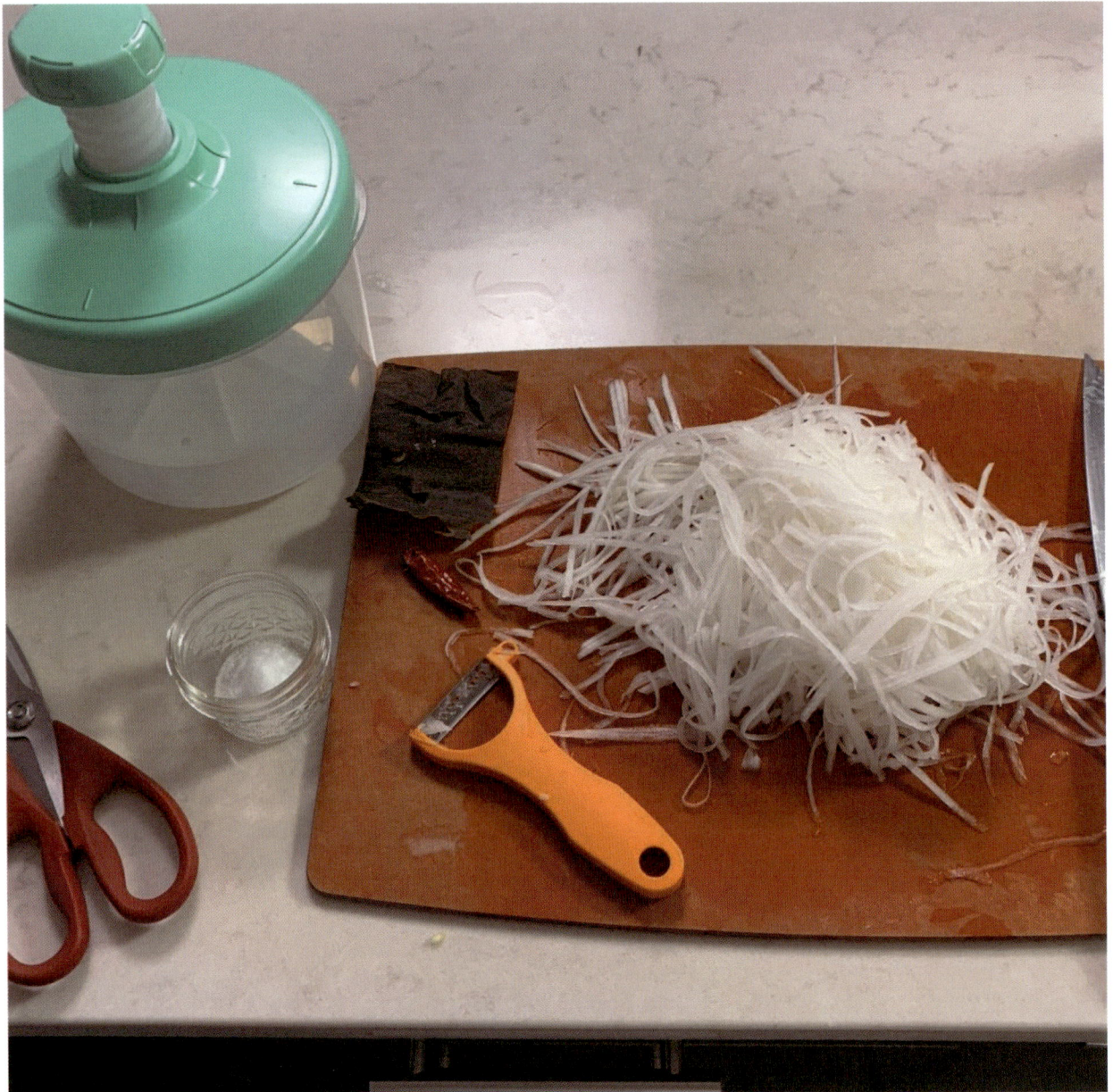

Ingredients for daikon otsukemono

Kyuri no Shougazuke
(Pickled cucumber with ginger)
生姜付け

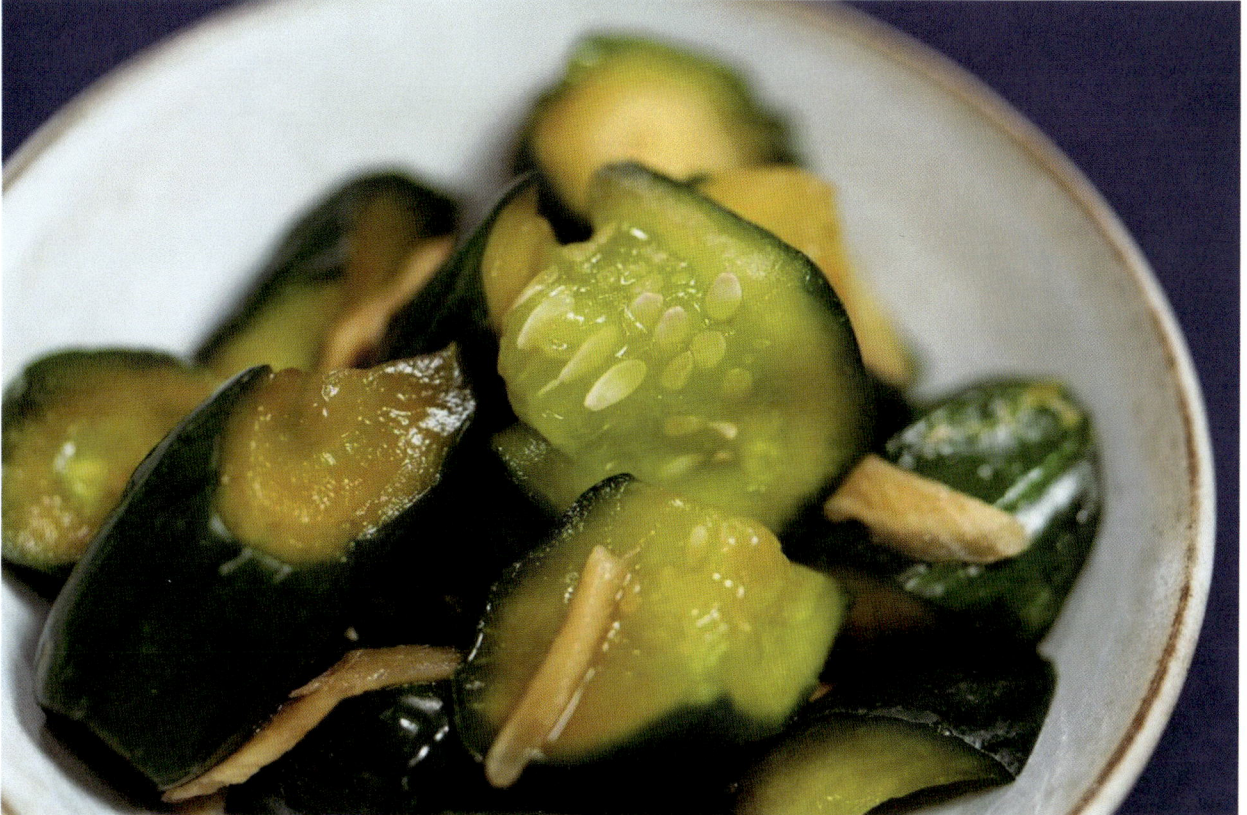

Shougazuke literally translated means to season with ginger.

There are many ways you can enjoy cucumber otsukemono. But pairing freshly cut ginger with cucumber and soy sauce is one of my favorite combinations. Especially during warm summer weather.

Using soy sauce rather than vinegar or salt also adds a richer flavor, without overpowering the flavor of the cucumber.

Makes 4-6 servings

Ingredients

- 1 lb Japanese cucumber, rangiri*
- 2 Tbsps fresh ginger, peeled and cut into matchsticks
- 4 g salt (1% total weight of cucumber)
- 2 Tbsps soy sauce
- 2 Tbsps mirin

Directions

1. Place the cut cucumber and ginger in a ziplock bag with the salt. Gently mix the bag so the salt is well distributed and allow to rest for 1 hour so water can be drawn out.
2. Strain the liquid and rinse the cucumber under cold running water to remove the salt.
3. Return to the bag and add in the soy sauce and mirin. Mix so all pieces are well coated with the pickling juice.
4. Allow to pickle overnight in the refrigerator.
5. The next day, remove the cucumber from the pickling juice.
6. Serve or use within 2-3 days.

Tips:

- *Rangiri, refer to page 39 for tips on this cutting technique.
- If you can't find Japanese cucumber, Persian cucumbers are a good alternative.
- Some cucumbers may have an unpleasant grassy and bitter flavor. If you're sensitive to it, shave off the skin closest to the end - the highest concentration of these compounds is near the tips.

Kyuri no Asazuke
(Pickled cucumber with soy sauce)
浅漬け

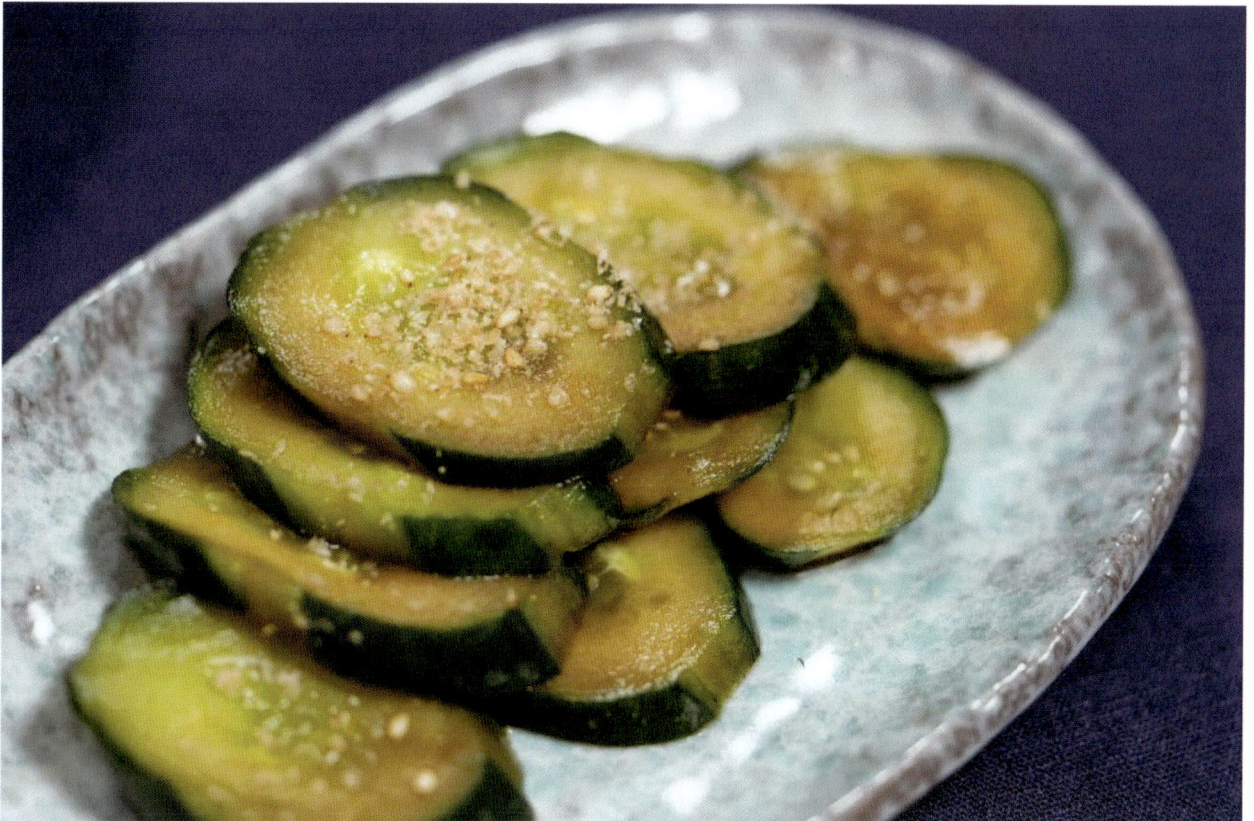

Asazuke literally translated means to 'shallow' seasoning. This type of otsukemono allow you to fully enjoy the natural flavors of the vegetables due to the light nature of the seasoning.

I vary the shapes every now and then but enjoy these most when sliced at an angle and topped with some toasted sesame seeds for a nice, nutty contrast.

Makes 4-6 servings

Ingredients

- 1 lb Japanese cucumber
- 3 Tbsps soy sauce
- 1 Tbsp mirin
- 2 in. square konbu

Directions

1. Peel 2-4 strips of the cucumber skin, lengthwise off of each cucumber. Then slice each piece ¼ in. thick at a 45-60 degree angle.
2. Lightly toast the konbu over a small open flame to soften, and cut into thin strips.
3. Add the cucumber, konbu strips, soy sauce and mirin to a ziplock bag.
4. Gently mix the bag to ensure all the pieces have come into contact with the pickling juice.
5. Allow to pickle in the refrigerator at least 2 hours.
6. Remove the cucumber from pickling juice and enjoy within 2-3 days.

Tips:

- For a different presentation style, cut the cucumber into other shapes such as rangiri as described on page 39. Simple round slices also work.
- Thinner cuts/slices of cucumbers will pickle quicker than thicker cuts (like rangiri). So if you're in a hurry, cut them on the thin side to save time.
- A good way to add another layer of flavor to both of these dishes is to use toasted and crushed sesame seeds or sesame oil.

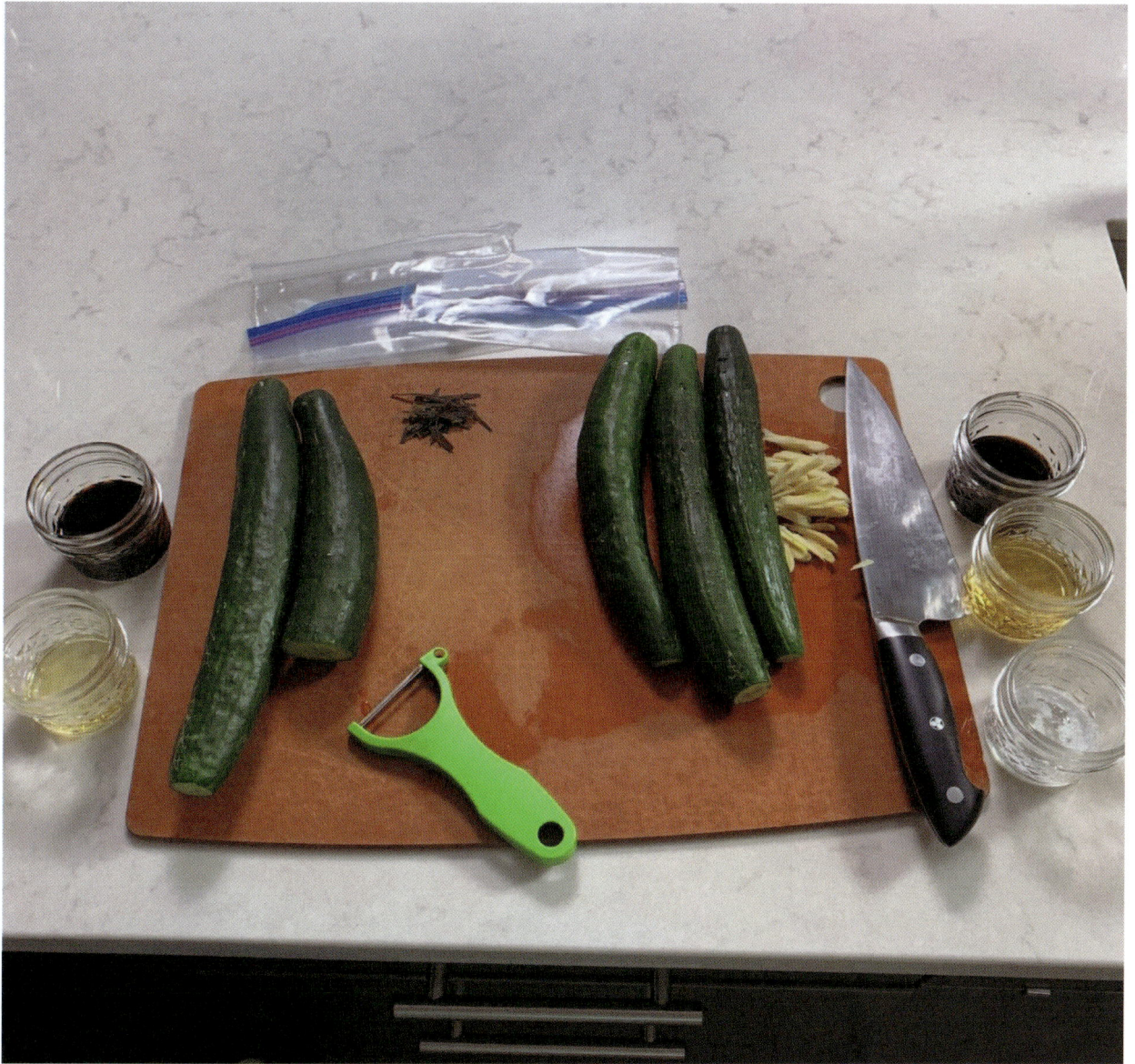

Ingredients for cucumber otsukemono

Gari (Pickled ginger)
ガリ

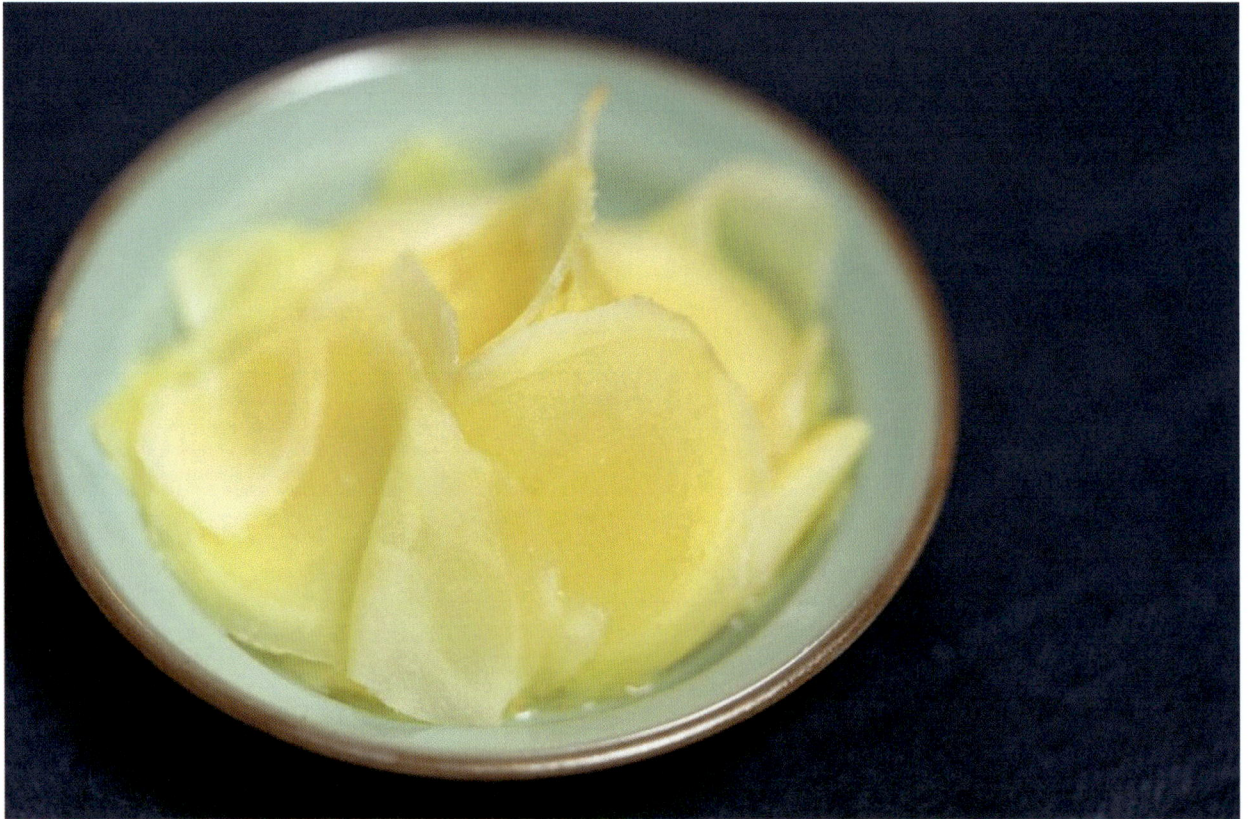

Ever since I began to like sushi, I've always enjoyed eating it with pickled ginger. Yes, can you believe there was a time when I didn't like sushi?

Like a lot of kids, I really didn't like sushi was when I was younger. What changed my mind were the canned tuna and mayo rolls with lettuce at Bristol Farms (a local market in Los Angeles, California).

Eventually, this led me to enjoy tekkamaki (鉄火巻き tuna roll), without wasabi at Noshizushi (a sushi restaurant in Hollywood).

I also thought I hated wasabi until I had the freshly grated rhizome in Japan.

And now wasabi is one of my favorite ways to spice things up. As you may know, wasabi can be used for many dishes aside from sushi, just like this pickled ginger can be used in a variety of ways too!

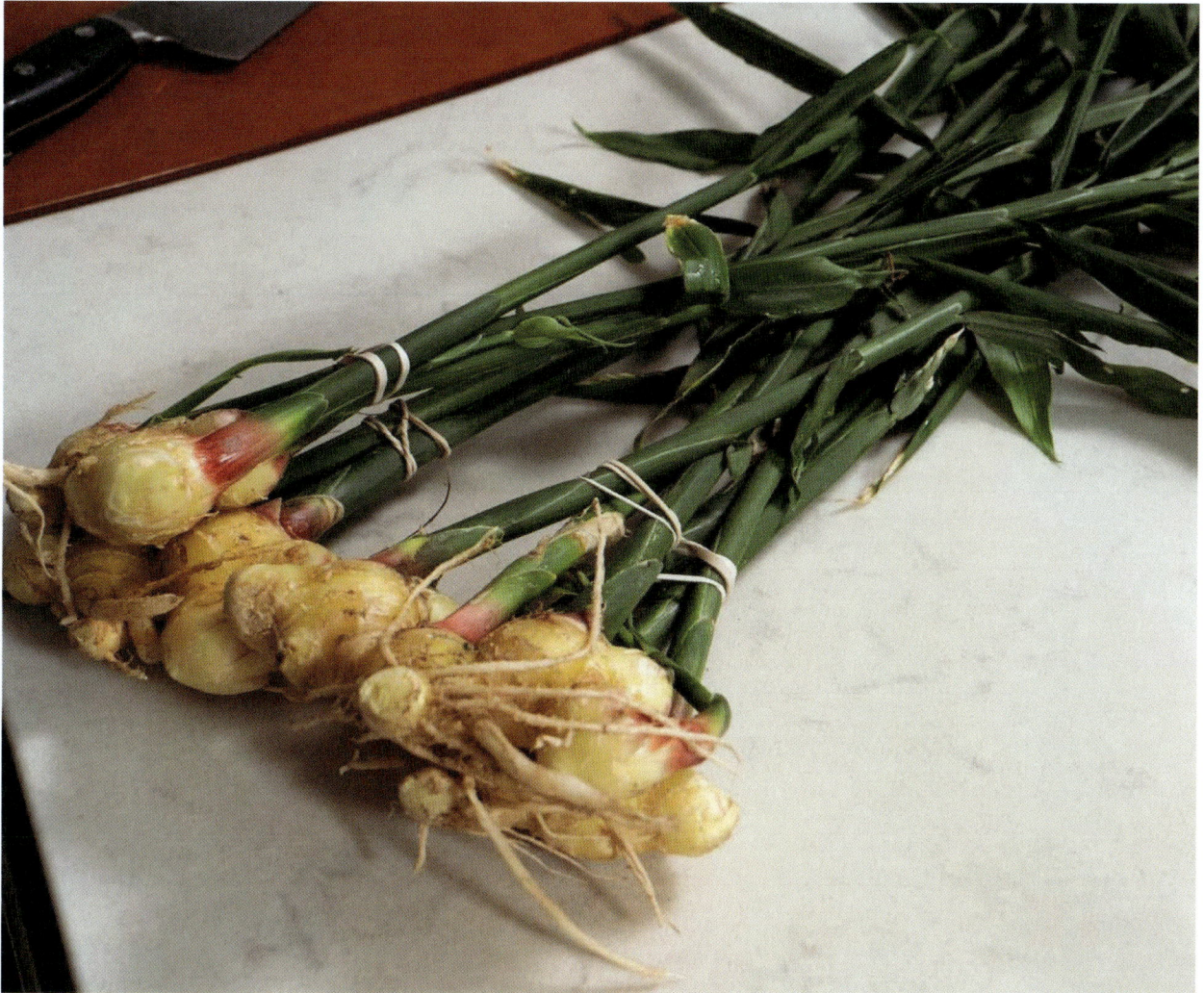

Fresh ginger stalks

Makes ~1 quart

Ingredients

- 1 lb. fresh ginger, skins peeled, roots removed and sliced thinly as possible (⅛ in. thick)
- ½ cup white sugar
- 1 ¼ tsp salt
- 2 cups rice vinegar

Directions

1. Prepare a medium pot with boiling water and a dash of salt.
2. Blanch the ginger slices for 1 minute.
3. Drain and allow to cool.
4. While cooling, heat a small sauce pan on medium low heat and dissolve the sugar and salt in the vinegar. Remove from the heat and allow to cool.
5. Once the ginger and vinegar mixture have cooled, mix them together in a quart jar or ziplock bag making sure each piece is has come into contact with the pickling juice.
6. Allow to pickle overnight in the refrigerator
7. Serve with sushi or any food you'd enjoy a pickled ginger flavor with!

Tips:

- The flavor and aroma is best in the first week, but it keeps for many months!
- When peeling the skin off the ginger, use the edge of a spoon to get in between any nubs more easily.
- Fresh ginger tends to be more fragile than dried and can break easily. If roots are attached, be gentle when pulling them off.
- If you'd like a natural pink color, include the pink/red areas near the green stalk.
  - Use a mandolin if you can. It'll save you time and give you perfectly even slices. On my PL8 mandolin, I use the thinnest setting for slicing. Visit alldayieat.com/go/bookresources for a product link.
- Make sure to slice the ginger the long way so you get nice long strips (it's also a lot less work!)
- If you can't find fresh, young ginger with fresh stalks and pink tips, that's okay! You can still use the dried brown kind, but note the ginger might end up being a bit more spicy. To offset this, add a bit more sugar.
- Consider growing your own ginger. It's easy to start from a dried piece and grows quickly. In a few months time, you'll have your own fresh supply ready to harvest!

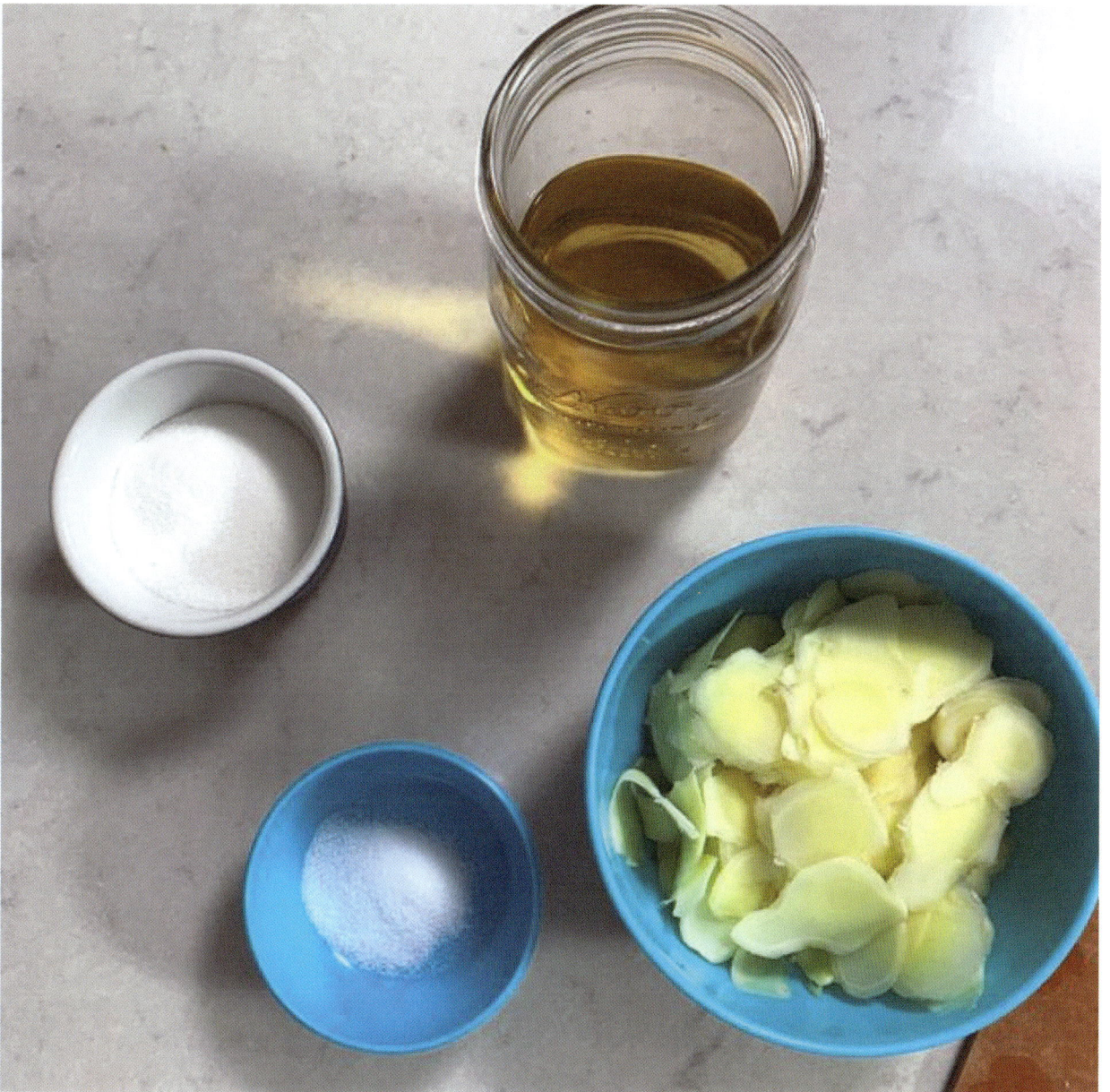

Ingredients for gari

Ninniku misozuke (Garlic pickled in miso)
ニンニク味噌漬け

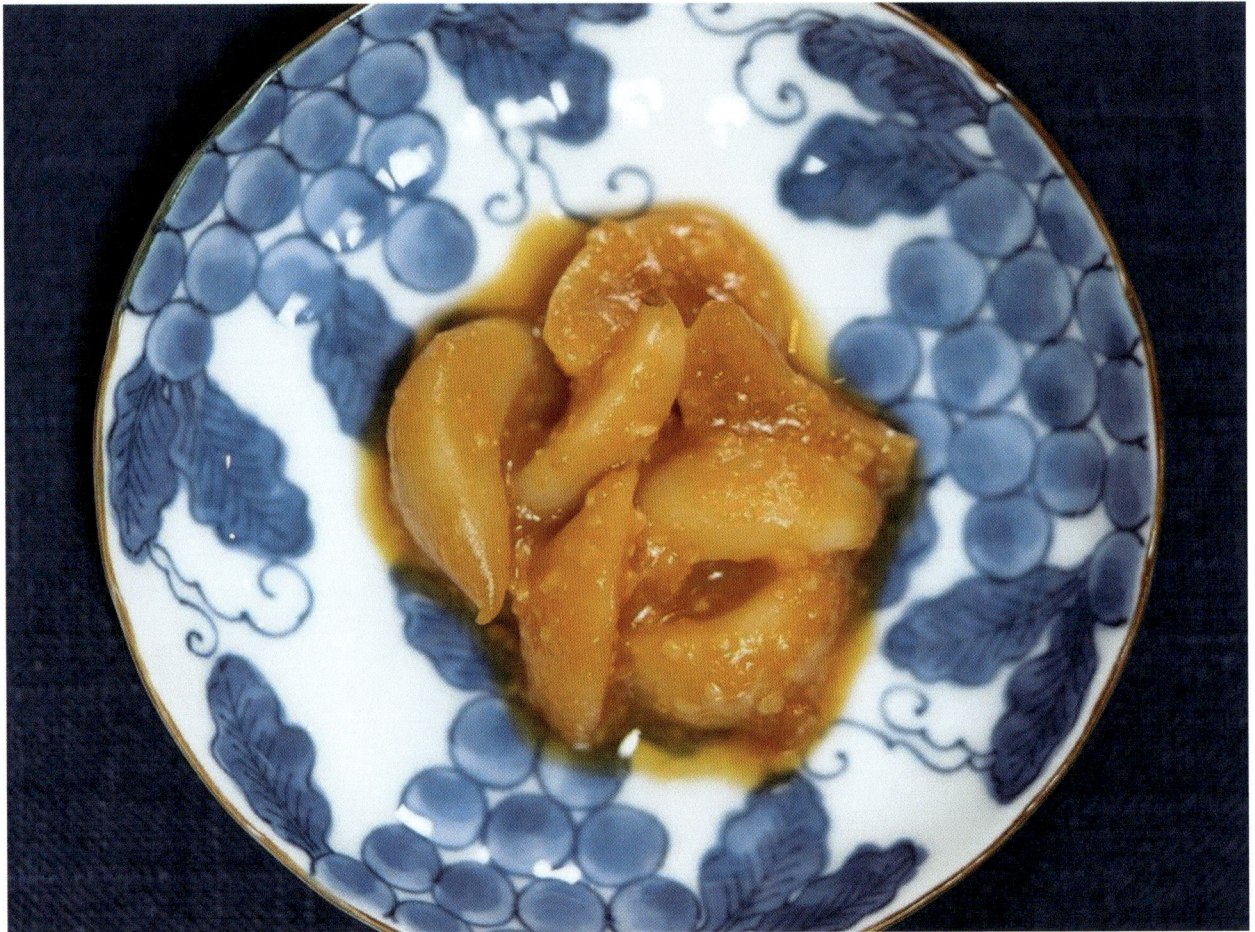

Garlic and miso are a wonderful combination and these pickled garlic cloves can be used in so many ways. Throw them in a dressing, in a stir-fry or just eat with plain rice.

If you love garlic and you love miso, you're gonna love these garlic pickles!

Makes ~1 cup

Ingredients

- ¼ lb. garlic cloves, skin peeled
- ¼ lb. red miso paste
- ¼ cup mirin

Directions

1. Prepare a small pot of boiling water and parboil the garlic for 1 minute.
2. Drain and pat dry.
3. Once cooled, transfer to a glass jar or ziplock bag and mix with the miso paste and mirin ensuring each piece is coated well.
4. Allow to pickle at least 2-3 days, then enjoy!

Tips:

- If using large garlic cloves, cut the pieces in half to increase surface area for the marinade and improve the flavor.
- In my opinion, the best flavor is about a week but it keeps for up to a month.
- Parboiling helps to take the spicy edge off the garlic but make sure not to overcook so the garlic doesn't get mushy.
- Miso tends to vary in flavor depending on the brand and the type. If you prefer saltier, stick with red miso. If you prefer sweeter lighter flavors try white miso. You can also try a 50/50 mixture of the two or add a tablespoon or two of sugar to the red miso mixture above.

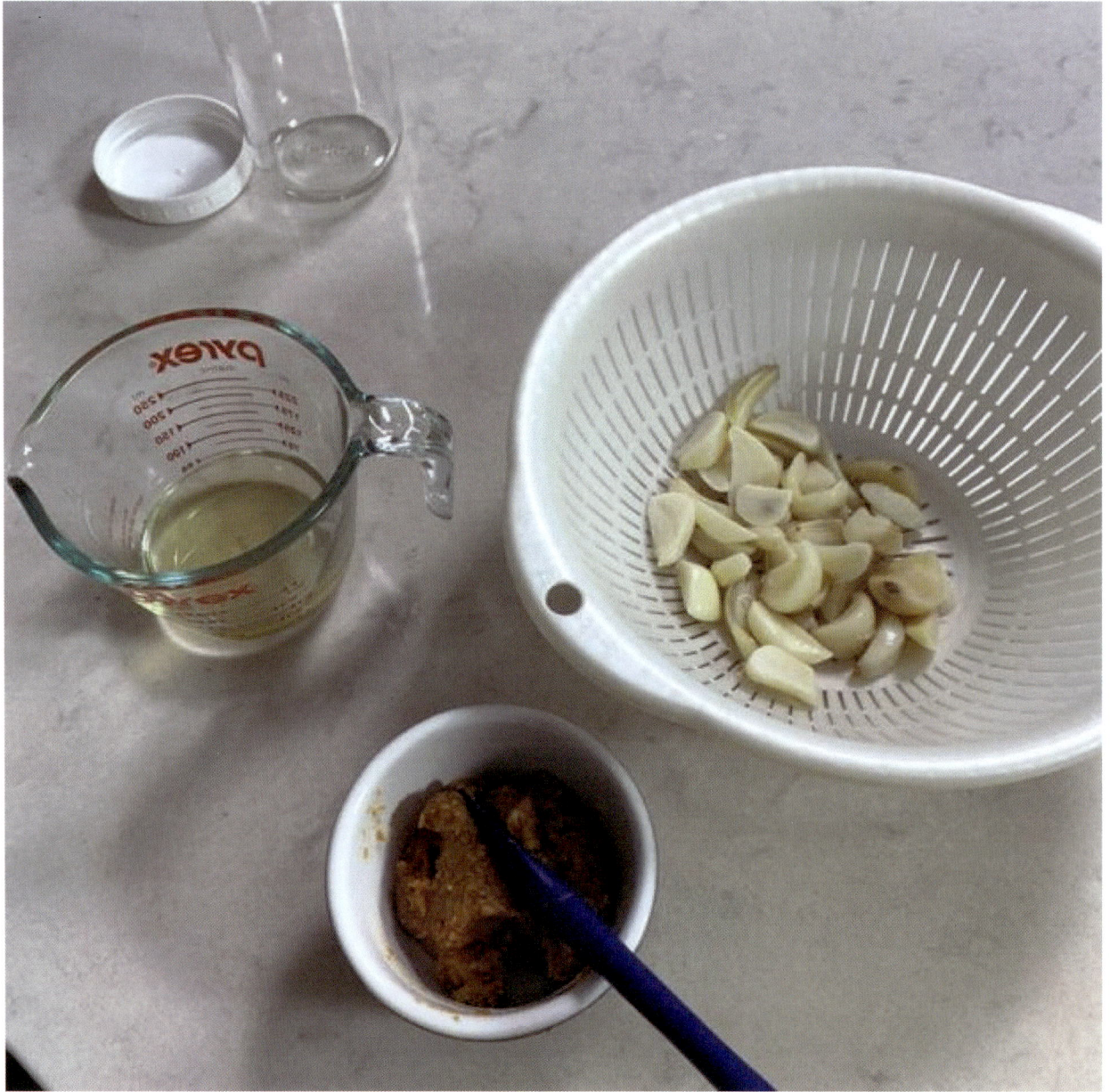

Ingredients for ninniku misozuke

Yasai Pasta (Vegetable pasta)

野菜パスタ

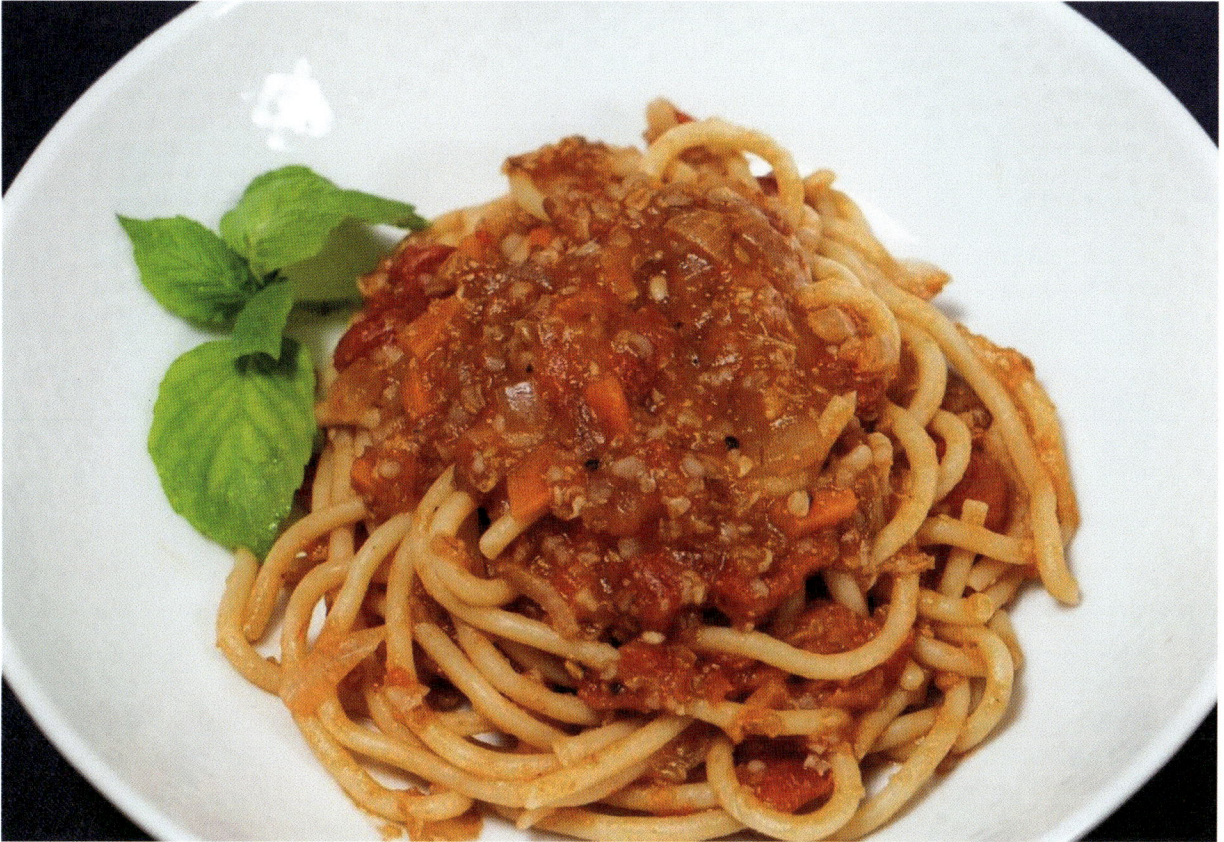

When I was growing up spaghetti and especially mitto sauce (ミートソース meat-sauce) spaghetti was one of my favorite dishes. And while there are many different recipes, this *meatless* version is one of my go-to dishes.

This recipe uses miso paste as the kakushiaji (隠し味 secret flavor). While you may think miso paste has a strong flavor, chances are you'd never know it was used in this dish! Hence the kakushiaji!

Miso paste adds plenty of umami (flavor enhancing compounds) that might just make this sauce one of your favorite ways to enjoy wafu pasta. Just thinking about this makes me hungry!

Makes 4 servings

Ingredients

- 1 lb. dried pici pasta, cooked until just before al dente*
- 1 cup carrots, chopped into quarters ¼ in. thick
- 1 cup onions, chopped ¼ in. thick
- 3-4 Tbsps extra-virgin olive oil
- 1 Tbsp ginger-garlic paste; alternatively, use ½ Tbsp minced ginger and ½ Tbsp minced garlic
- ¼ cup red wine, (such as a Cabernet)
- ¼ cup red miso paste
- 1 - 1 ½ cups bulgur wheat, cooked and drained
- 28 oz can whole tomatoes
- Freshly cracked black pepper

Toppings - freshly chopped Italian parsley, Italian basil, Kaiware daikon (radish sprouts), shiso (perilla), green onions, freshly cracked black pepper

Directions

1. Cook your pasta in salted water until just before al dente. Then drain, reserving ½ cup cooking pasta water to thin sauce, if desired. Cover the pasta and set aside until sauce is ready.
2. Using a large sauté pan on medium high heat, add olive oil, carrots and onions and a dash of salt. Cook for 4-5 minutes until they begin to brown.
3. Add ginger-garlic paste and cook for 1 minute until fragrant.
4. Add in miso paste, red wine, tomatoes, and bulgur. Cook uncovered, stirring occasionally for another 10-15 minutes until the alcohol has evaporated.
5. Add reserved pasta water to thin the sauce, if desired

To serve

1. For one person, take ¼ lb. cooked pasta and add to the pot with the sauce. Cook on low heat for about 30-45 seconds and then serve! If cooking for multiple people, add all at once and mix until sauce evenly coats the noodles.
2. Top with desired toppings and enjoy!

Tips:

Perfecting your pasta

- * Pici is a thick pasta noodle that offers a nice bite and pairs well with this tomato sauce. Alternatives to pici include bucatini or spaghetti.
- When buying dried pasta, look for pasta that has a rough texture (almost looks like dust or powder). That irregular surface texture helps the sauce cling to the pasta. Rustichella is brand worth trying. Visit alldayieat.com/go/bookresources for a product link.
- When making pasta, salt your water to add flavor to your pasta. I use about 1 ½ tablespoons in 12 cups of water to cook 1 lb. of pasta.
- By not cooking the pasta all the way to al dente, you'll be able to finish cooking it in the pasta sauce. Doing this helps the pasta absorb flavor from the sauce as it finishes cooking. Try this and see if you can notice a difference!
- Adjust the seasoning to your tastes. Add a few teaspoons of sugar or honey to sweeten it. Add a dash of salt, shiokouji, or soy sauce to make it more savory.
- If you enjoy thin pasta sauces, use the reserved pasta water to thin the sauce. On the contrary, if you like very thick sauces, simmer an extra 20-30 minutes stirring occasionally to thicken it.
- The sauce freezes well so you can easily double or triple the quantity for a quick and tasty meal at a later date.

Variations worth exploring

- Substitute or add a small handful of vegetables. Okra, eggplant, zucchini, and fresh Japanese mushrooms (enoki, maitake, shiitake, shimeji) are tasty ways to add additional flavors and textures. Cook with the carrots or onions if using.
- Substitute the bulgur grain with a similar amount of cooked farro or chickpeas.
- Try using Italian tomatoes which tend to be sweeter and a little smoother in flavor, as compared to American grown tomatoes.

Miso potato itame (Miso-glazed potatoes)

味噌ポテト炒め

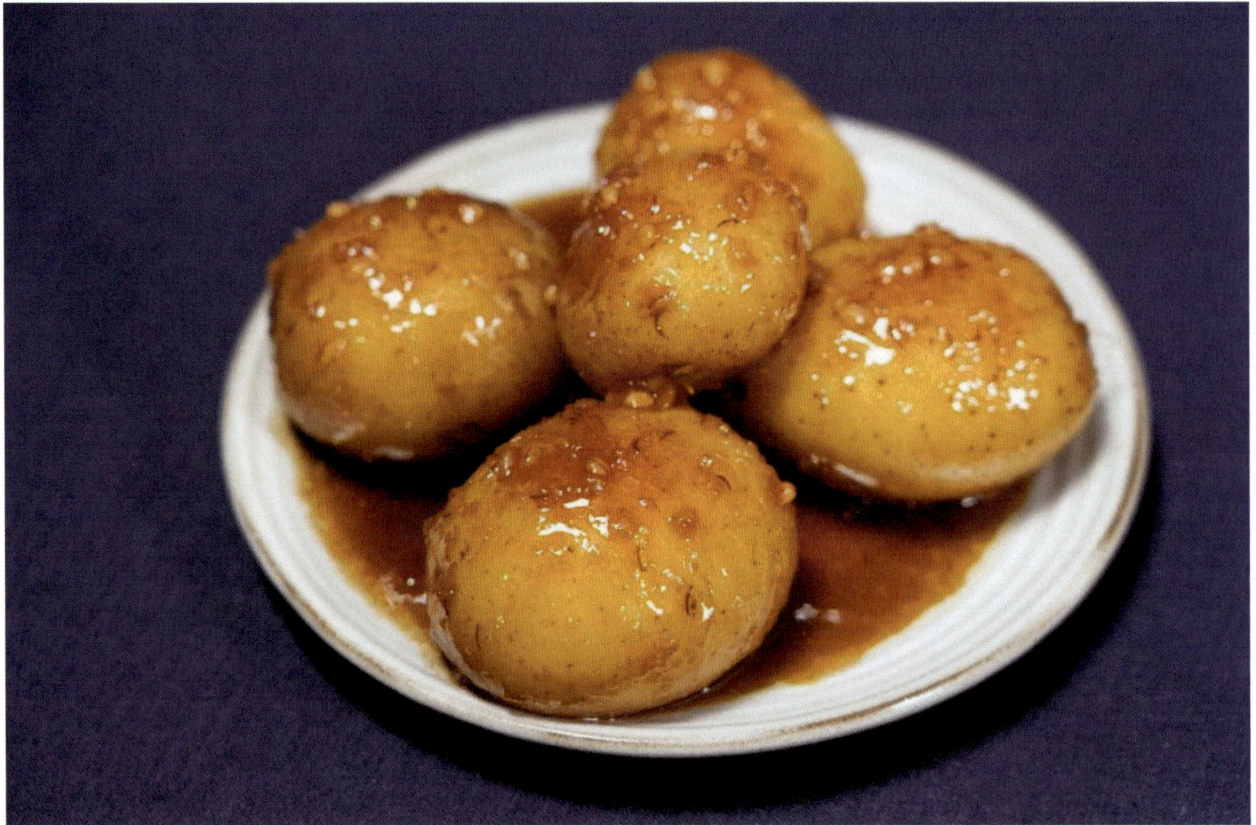

When I was a child, my parents and relatives teased me for liking potatoes more than rice. I still love potatoes and aside from my homemade oven fries, I enjoy baking them, making a salad with them and using them in soups.

Because potatoes can be starchy and have a lot of body, they usually need a strong seasoning.

If you haven't yet tried seasoning potatoes with miso, this might soon become one of your favorite ways to enjoy them.

Makes 6-8 servings

Ingredients

- 1 lb. Yukon gold potatoes, boiled
- 3-4 Tbsps extra-virgin olive oil
- ½ cup konbu shiitake dashi
- 2 Tbsps red miso paste, (I used barley)
- 2 Tbsps soy sauce
- 1 Tbsp sugar
- 6 Tbsps mirin

Toppings - sesame oil or toasted and ground sesame seeds

Directions

1. Cook the potatoes in a pot of water until you can easily pierce them with a chopstick. Drain and set aside.
2. Using a large sauté pan on medium heat, add the olive oil and potatoes, brown both sides of the potatoes (2-3 minutes per side).
3. Meanwhile, combine the dashi with the miso, soy sauce, sugar, and mirin. Make sure to break apart any clumps of miso paste and set aside.
4. Once both sides of the potatoes have browned, add in the dashi mixture and cook until the liquid is reduced, rotating potatoes 2-3 times while reducing.
5. After liquid has reduced to a thick, gravy-like consistency, serve warm.

Tips:

- I recommend using Yukon gold potatoes for the best texture. They're rich and creamy, and cook relatively quickly compared to larger potatoes like russet.
- This miso-based glaze is filled with a ton of umami and will allow you to enjoy a classic Japanese flavor, very reminiscent of osembei (お煎餅 grilled rice crackers seasoned with soy sauce).
- The great thing about the glaze is that it can be used for other sautéed vegetables too. I like it with sautéed or steamed green beans and asparagus the most. Japanese eggplant and green bell peppers are another favorite and work well with this sauce too. You can even use it for onigiri (おにぎり rice balls).
- If you're in the mood for something sweeter, top a baked Japanese sweet potato with this glaze for a tasty alternative to regular potatoes!

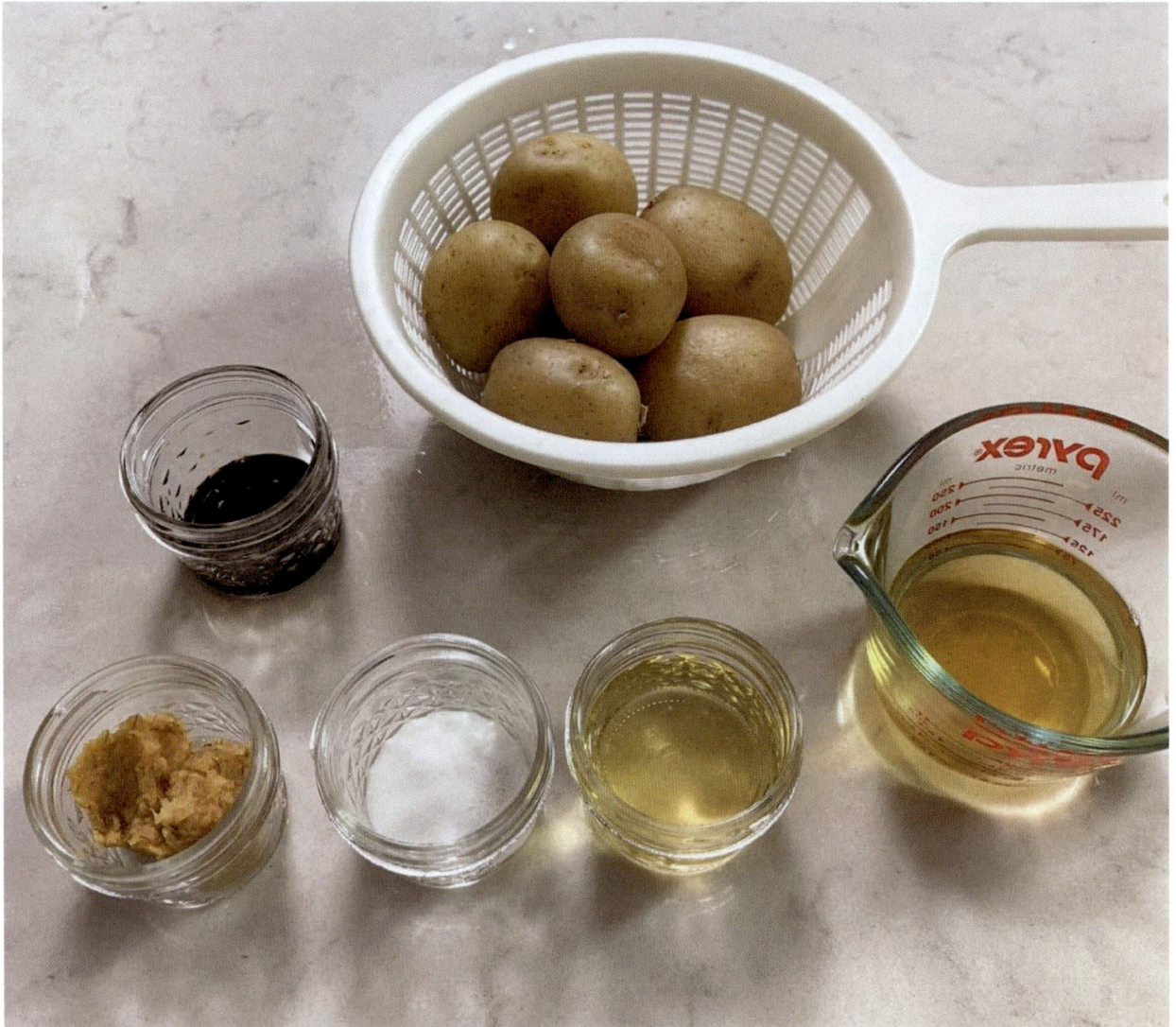

Ingredients for miso-glazed potatoes

Misonikomi Udon (Miso simmered udon)

味噌煮込みうどん

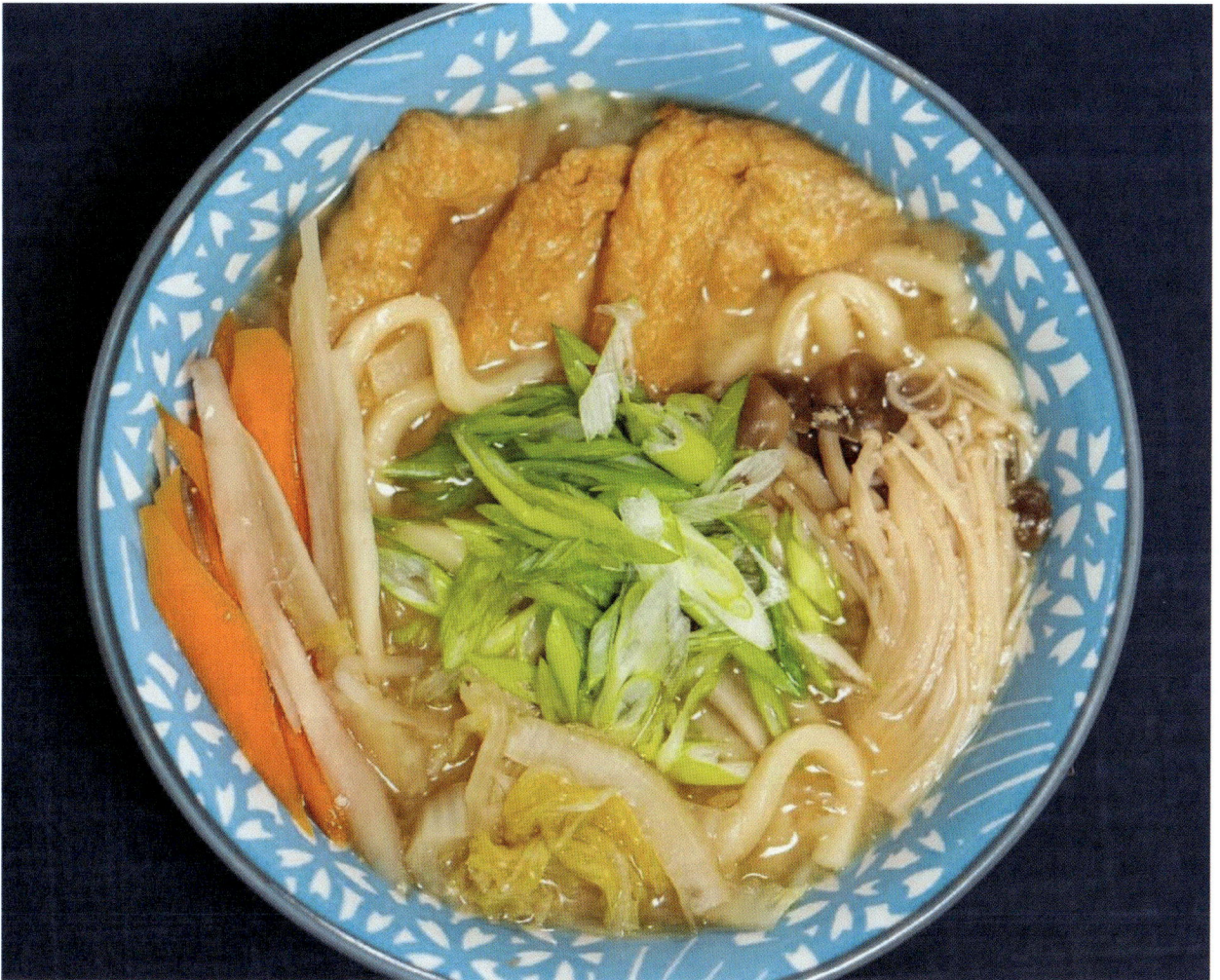

Is it just me or does it seem like udon noodles aren't as popular as ramen? I wonder why...

Anyway, if I owned and operated an udon noodle restaurant, this is one dish I'd have on the menu. Many noodles dishes call for something called mentsuyu (麺つゆ noodle soup base).

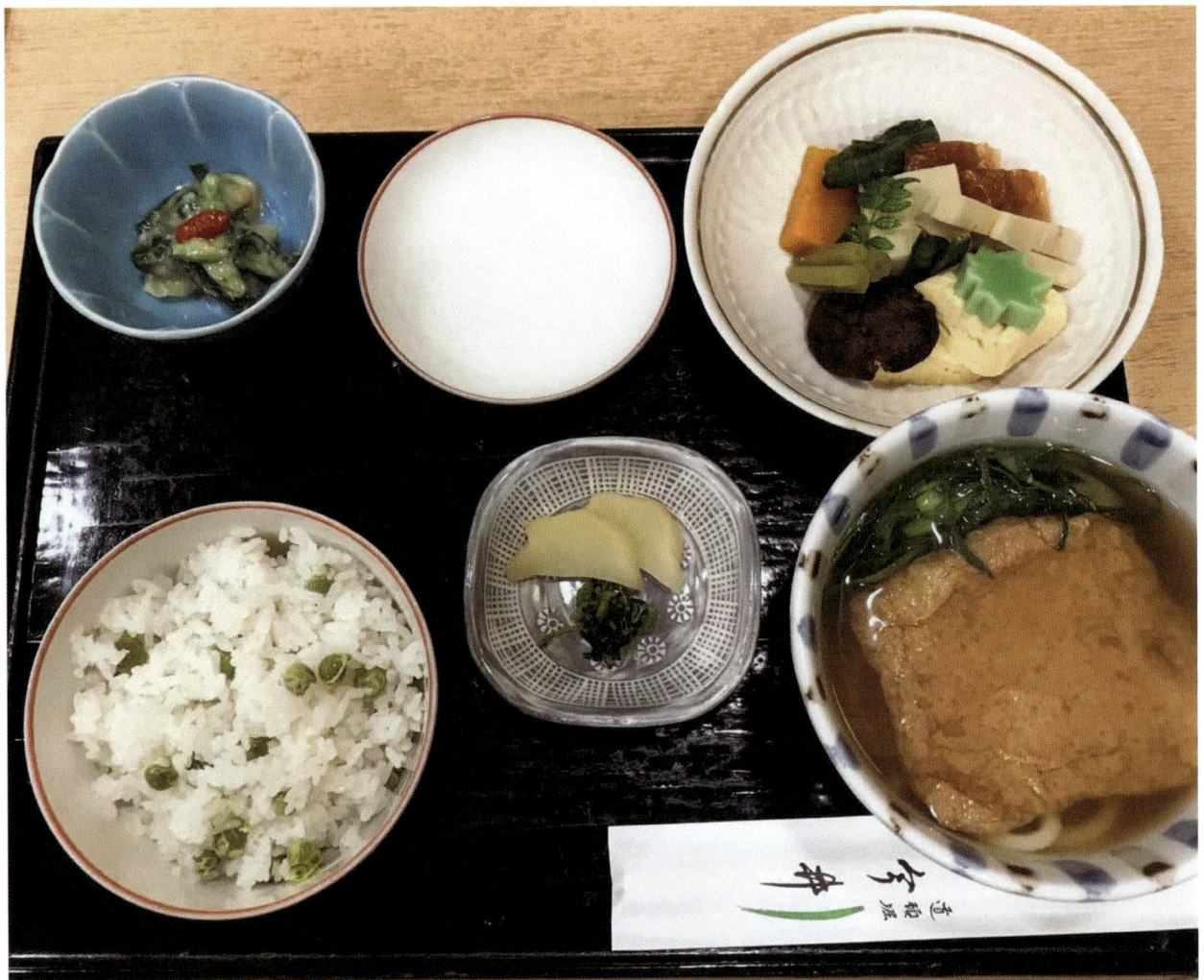

Kitsune udon teishoku (set meal)

Chances are if you've had soba or udon you've eaten or used mentsuyu before. But If you're in the mood for something different, this is a good alternative that's well worth making!

The best part?

You can rotate the types of miso used for different flavors as well as the vegetables depending on what you've got on hand. This means endless flavor and texture combinations and a dish you might enjoy on a very regular basis.

Makes 4-5 servings

Ingredients

For the soup base

- 5 cups konbu shiitake dashi
- ¼ cup mirin
- 6-8 Tbsps red miso paste

Vegetables

- 1 bunch udon noodles per person, cooked per pack directions
- 1-2 carrots, peeled and cut sasagaki*
- ½ piece gobo, skin removed and cut sasagaki*
- ½ onion, thinly sliced
- 1 bunch green onion, cut at a 60-degree angle into 1-2 in. pieces
- 4-6 leaves napa cabbage, cut into 1 in. pieces
- 1 pack aburaage, (deep fried tofu skins); or 1 block firm tofu, drained
- 1 pack enoki mushrooms, bottoms trimmed; or 6-8 pieces dashigara shiitake (leftover shiitake from making dashi)

Toppings - chopped green onions, mitsuba (Japanese parsley), ichimi or shichimi red pepper

Directions

1. Using a large pot or dutch oven on medium heat, combine the dashi with the mirin and bring to a gentle simmer and evaporate the alcohol.
2. Add the miso paste, the vegetables, and the udon noodles and cook partially covered for 4-8 minutes.
3. Once vegetables have softened and noodles are cooked through, it's ready to serve!

Tips:

- *For gobo and carrots, refer to the okara misoshiru tips on page 35.
- Look for udon noodles without salt, as the broth will have plenty of seasoning from the miso. Or if you're up to it, make them yourself. Homemade udon noodles are some of the easiest noodles to make.

Getting the best flavor

- If you'd like a little more flavor from your vegetables, brown them in a sauté pan with some olive oil first.
- To add more flavor to the noodles cook them in the broth, rather than boiling separately and then adding. And it's one less step ☺
- For the richest flavor - try to use red miso that's primarily made with soy beans. The following three miso pastes in particular have equally rich and unique flavors:
  - hacchou miso 八丁味噌
  - shinshu miso 信州味噌 (sweeter)
  - akadashi 赤だし (contains fish)
- Because the red miso soup base has a very robust flavor, this is another versatile dish with which you can use a variety of vegetables as you would with nabe (hot pot).

Kanten (Agar)
寒天

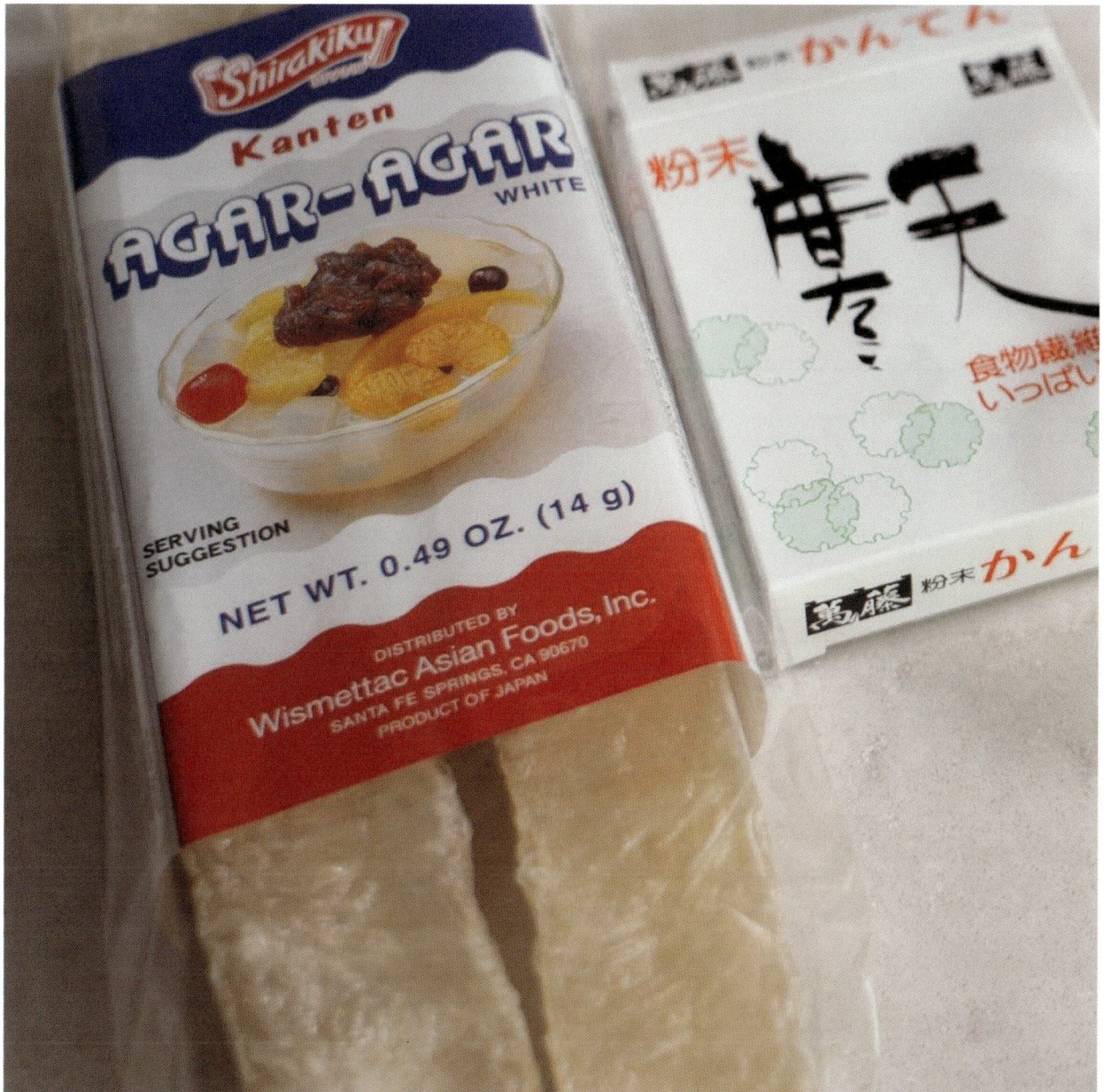

It's said that kanten was discovered by accident in the 1600's by a Kyoto innkeeper named Minoya Tarozaemon. He made a lot of tokoroten (ところてん

jelly noodle dish) that's traditionally made with the tengusa (天草 dried seaweed). Because it was somewhat labor-intensive to make from scratch, historically, this dish was reserved for the wealthy.

Although kanten is made in Japan there are other countries that also produce the product. Agar has always been a staple in dessert-making in many Asian countries so there many other variations of kanten-like desserts and dishes.

In case you were wondering, there are a few differences between agar, kanten and gelatin. Agar (agar-agar) comes from a type of red algae from the genus Gracilaria, while kanten is made from a smaller genus of red algae called Gelidiales. Because they're similar, you can substitute them using a 1:1 ratio.

But comparing agar or kanten to gelatin is a different story. Gelatin is made from the collagen that is found in the skin and bones of animals. Gelatin is mainly produced by boiling down these animal parts to a gel.

To many foodies, the main difference between kanten and gelatin would be the texture of the food they're used in. Gelatin generally has a softer more delicate texture or mouth feel while kanten is firmer or has more 'bite'.

One additional benefit of using kanten over gelatin is that kanten doesn't melt at room temperature. This would be ideal if you're thinking of bringing jelly-like dessert to a potluck.

Being plant-based, kanten naturally contains dietary fiber which only comes from plant sources. Dietary fiber helps eliminate cholesterol and other non-beneficial things from your gut. And another plus is that it has almost no calories!

Kanten is basically dried up, processed seaweed but it comes in many forms.

The most convenient forms that you can buy in the market are the kanten sticks and kanten powder. Outside of Japan, other forms of kanten such as flakes and raw tengusa are quite rare.

Like gelatin or agar-agar, if you've used them before, it's main use is to solidify a liquid.

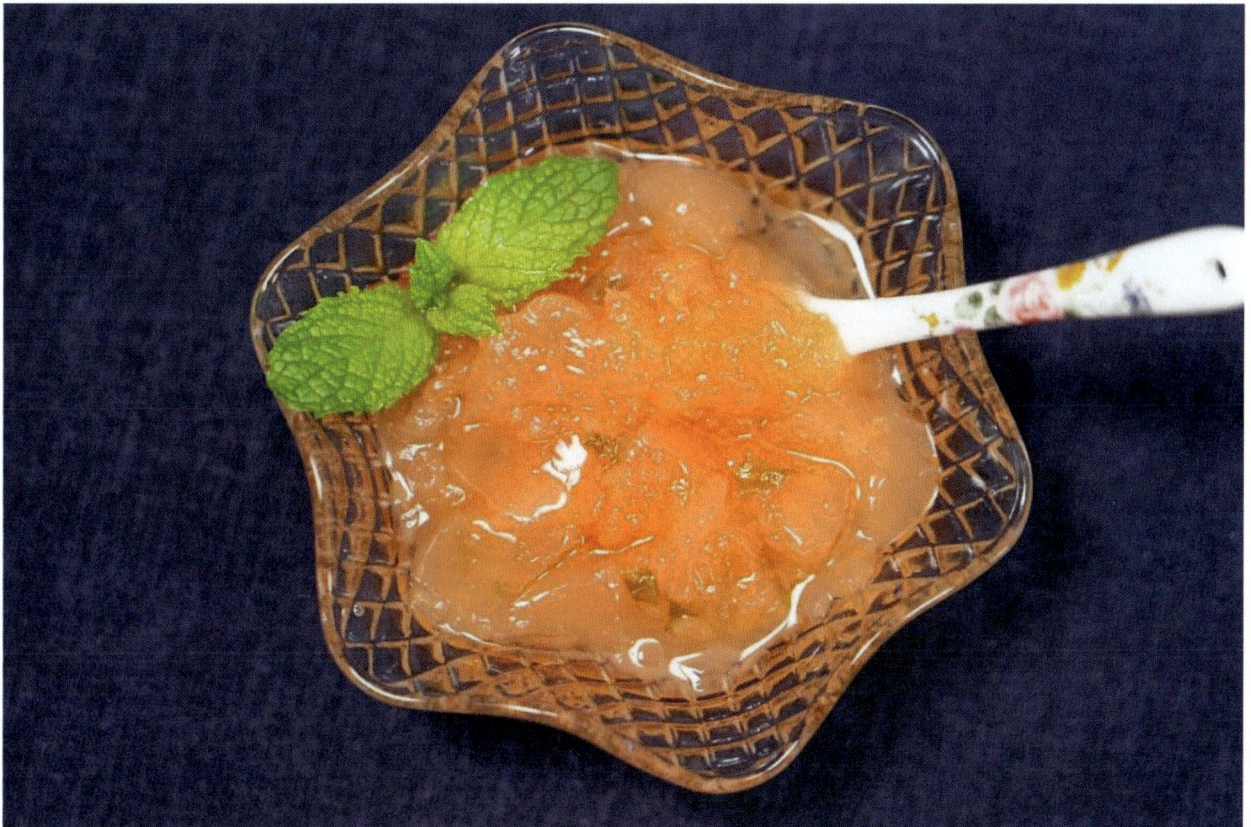

Grapefruit zeri (ゼリー jelly) with kanten

Tokoroten (Agar noodles)
ところてん

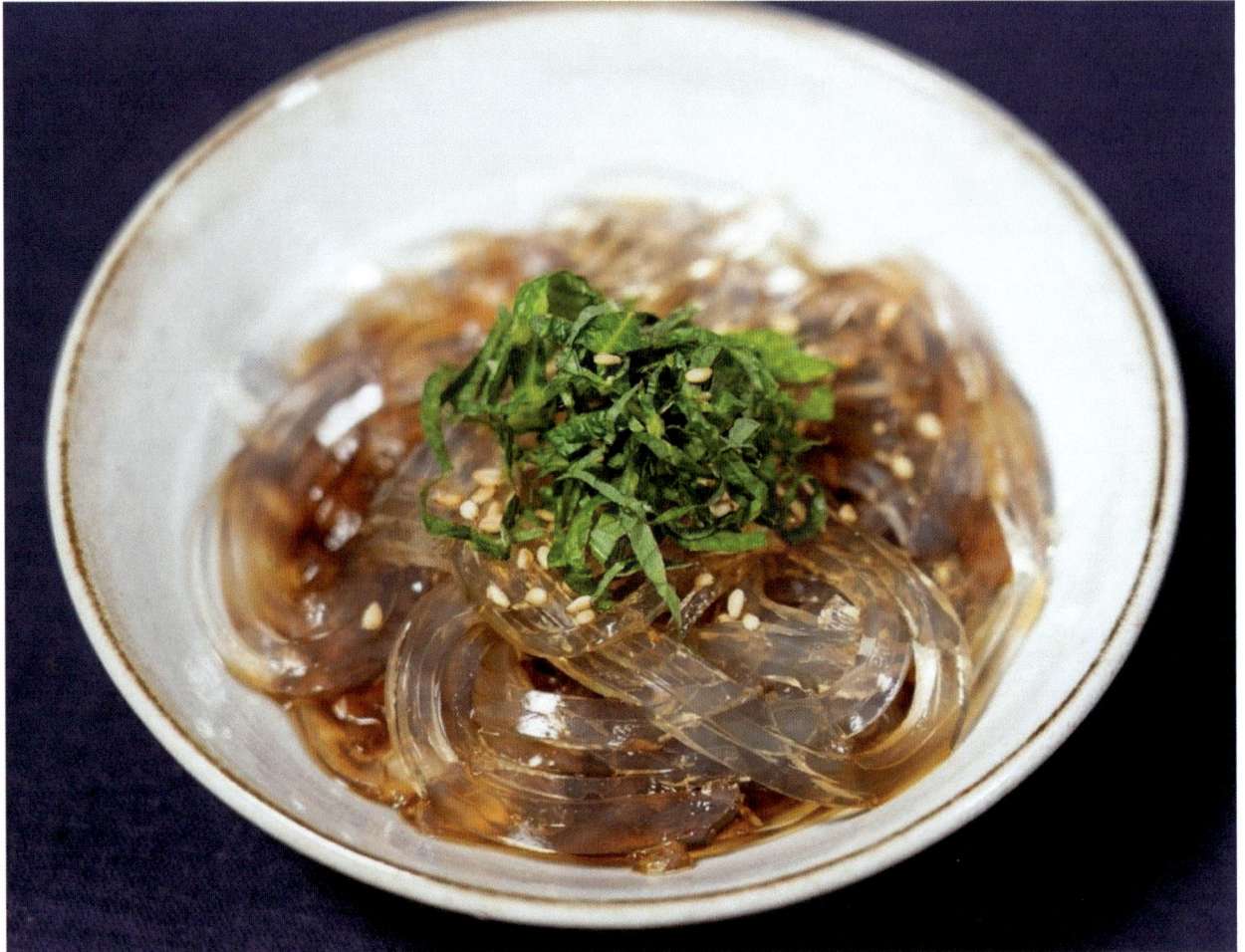

Tokoroten are noodles made from kanten. It makes for a light and refreshing snack when you're in the mood for something tasty and light.

With virtually no flavor of their own, they can be seasoned in many different ways, both savory and sweet. On the next page you'll learn how to make sanbaizu, which is a vinegar based sauce that's the perfect way to season these noodles.

Makes 4-6 servings

Ingredients

For the tokoroten

- 4 g powdered kanten
- 1 ¾ cups water

For the sanbaizu (三杯酢 three sake cup vinegar)

- 2 Tbsps soy sauce
- 2 Tbsps nikitta mirin, (mirin with alcohol cooked off in the microwave for 20-30 secs)
- 2 Tbsps rice vinegar

  Toppings – Shiso (perilla), freshly toasted sesame seeds (whole or ground), a dash of sesame oil (optional)

Directions

1. Using a medium size sauce pan, add the water and the powdered kanten.
2. Stir with a whisk until there are no clumps and bring to a gentle boil.
3. Simmer for 3-5 minutes (per packet directions).
4. Remove from heat, transfer to a flat, square or rectangular temperature-safe container and cover.
5. Once cool to the touch, place in the refrigerator for 2-3 hours to set.
6. Using a tokorotentsuki (tokoroten device), cut a piece to fit in the hole and push through. Repeat for desired quantity.
7. Alternatively, use a chef's knife to cut the kanten into ¼ in. thick rectangles, and then cut the rectangles into ¼ in. x ¼ in. thick noodles.
8. Serve on a small plate and top with sanbaizu and desired toppings.

Tips:

- If you can't find powdered kanten, substitute 4 grams of powdered kanten with:
  - 4 grams agar-agar
  - ½ stick kanten; learn how to prepare stick kanten at alldayieat.com/go/bookresources
- For a firmer texture, use less water. For a softer texture, use a bit more. Adjust the water 2-3 tablespoons at a time to see what you like best.
- Substitute the shiso with kaiware daikon (radish sprouts), chopped green onion, kimchi, pickled ginger, freshly grated ginger, or wasabi
- For a sweet alternative, use kuromitsu (黒蜜 black Okinawan sugar syrup). Okinawa is a major producer of this type of sugar in Japan. Visit alldayieat.com/go/bookresources for a product link.
- This is a dish you'll want to eat cool or chilled and is especially refreshing in the summer, thanks to the light, vinegar-based seasoning and lightness of the tokoroten.
- The sanbaizu can be used to season other foods such as a cucumber and wakame (seaweed) salad or even tofu.

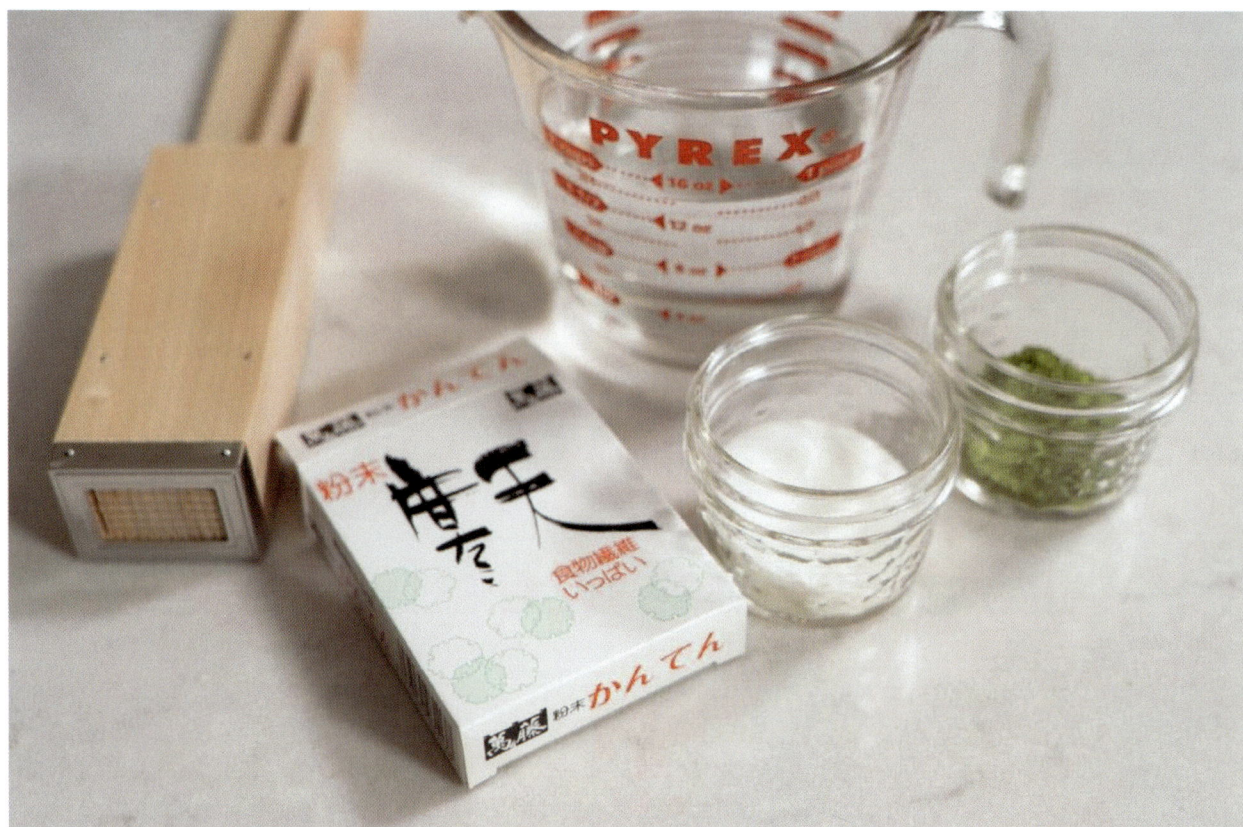

Tokorotentsuki (ところてん突き top left)

Thank you!

Omedetougozaimasu! おめでとうございます!

Congratulations! You made it to the end! I just wanted to acknowledge your achievement and for taking the time to invest in yourself with plant-based Japanese cooking.

You know I'm all about baby steps and by trying some of the recipes in this book, you've gained momentum and confidence to expand your horizons in plant-based cooking and eating.

I'm grateful to have your support and also for the opportunity to serve you.

I hope you've enjoyed this culinary journey to Japan and that you one day get a chance to visit!

Japan is a unique and endlessly fascinating country. And whenever you make Japanese food in your kitchen, perhaps it'll bring back fond memories for you, such as your travels there or the delicious food you've eaten.

Wishing you the best of luck and continued success in life and all your cooking endeavors! Ganbattene (頑張ってね you got this!)

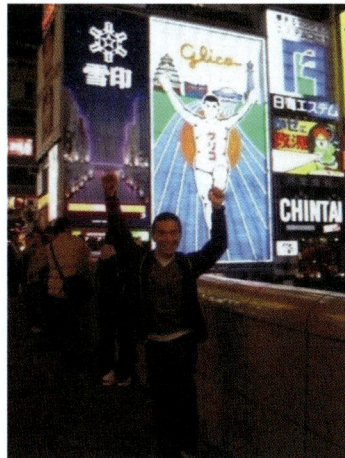

-Pat

Your next steps

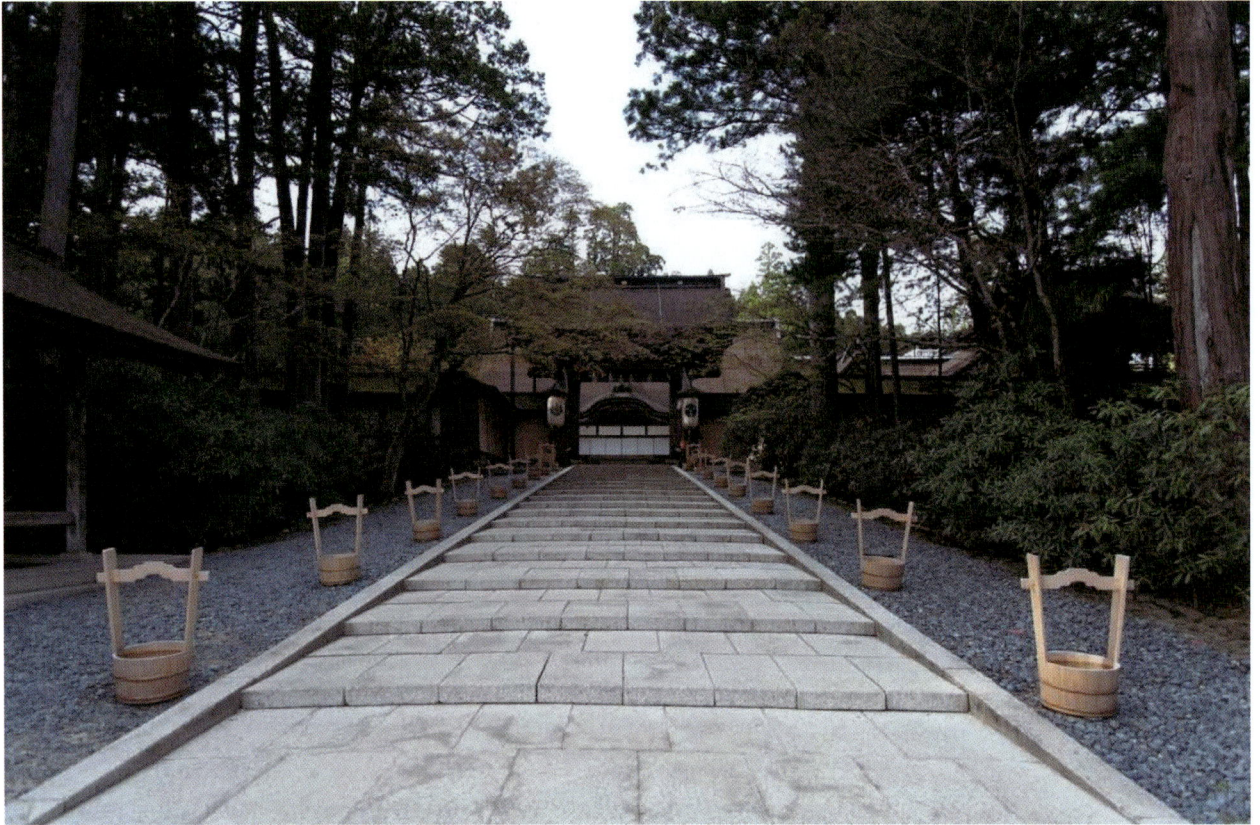

Entrance to a temple, Mount Koya, Japan

1. Take action

With action comes clarity. You'll gain invaluable, firsthand experience by cooking yourself, rather than reading or watching someone else do it.
With experience comes skill and confidence.
If others can cook plant-based Japanese food, so can you!

Repetition is the mother of all learning. The more you cook, the more efficient and better you'll get (and that includes your intuition too).

2. Share your progress

We'd love to feature your photos and posts about plant-based Japanese cooking. Just include the hashtag #yatta when posting photos and videos on your favorite social network.

Share a photo of you with the book, your favorite line or passage, or any ideas that struck you that might inspire others to follow in your footsteps.

3. Participate in the community

As you cook plant-based Japanese food, you'll probably come up with questions or ideas you'd love to get feedback on. Having a community of like-minded people who know what you're going through and can relate to road blocks or frustrations you face will make all the difference in your cooking adventures.

Chances are, if you have a question, others do too. So, it's an act of generosity on your part to ask it! There are no dumb questions. The dumb thing is not asking or assuming.

Ask and you shall receive!

Thank you for your active participation and contributions to the community! (Request access at **alldayieat.com/go/community**)

4. Enjoy the journey

Life was never meant to be a struggle. Looking back, I've come to realize I used to be a pretty serious person. And I used to get upset when things didn't happen the way I wanted them to. Whether it was in the form of a failed dish or a simple mistake of getting on a long-distance non-stop train without first checking to see where it was going. (Yes, this really happened.) There is beauty and something good to be found in any situation, you just might have to look for it a bit.

Seek and you will find!

5. Let me know your thoughts

As you probably know, feedback is essential when it comes to providing valuable content and making things better for next time. In Japanese, there's this term you may have heard of kaizen (改善 to improve or redo for the better). And that's what I set out to do each and every time I release my creations into the world. If you could, please share your feedback in a short 3 question survey at **alldayieat.com/go/jccbooksurvey**

6. Check out the resources page

For video tips on Japanese cooking techniques, ingredients, cooking supplies, helpful books, and other resources, visit **alldayieat.com/go/bookresources**

7. Consider joining the Japanese Cooking Club

If you're looking for step-by-step video cooking lessons, resources, and want to connect with like-minded people who are also committed to the plant-based lifestyle. The Japanese Cooking Club is for you. To find out more visit **alldayieat.com/go/joinjcc**

Knock (gently) and the door will open for you!

Acknowledgements

This cookbook and all that I've shared over the past few years would not have been possible without many people who have helped and guided me along the way.

My parents especially, Cathy and Yo, who've always been there to support me.

My younger brother and sister, Sean and Evelyn for feedback on what I could do better.

Emi, my girlfriend who's always eating up the food I cook and replacing it with an endless stream of cooking ideas.

My core team: Mariphel, Gelo, Karina, Sarah, and Ira for all the behind-the-scenes work you do to make the Japanese Cooking Club and all day I eat like a shark possible.

Thank you.

About the author

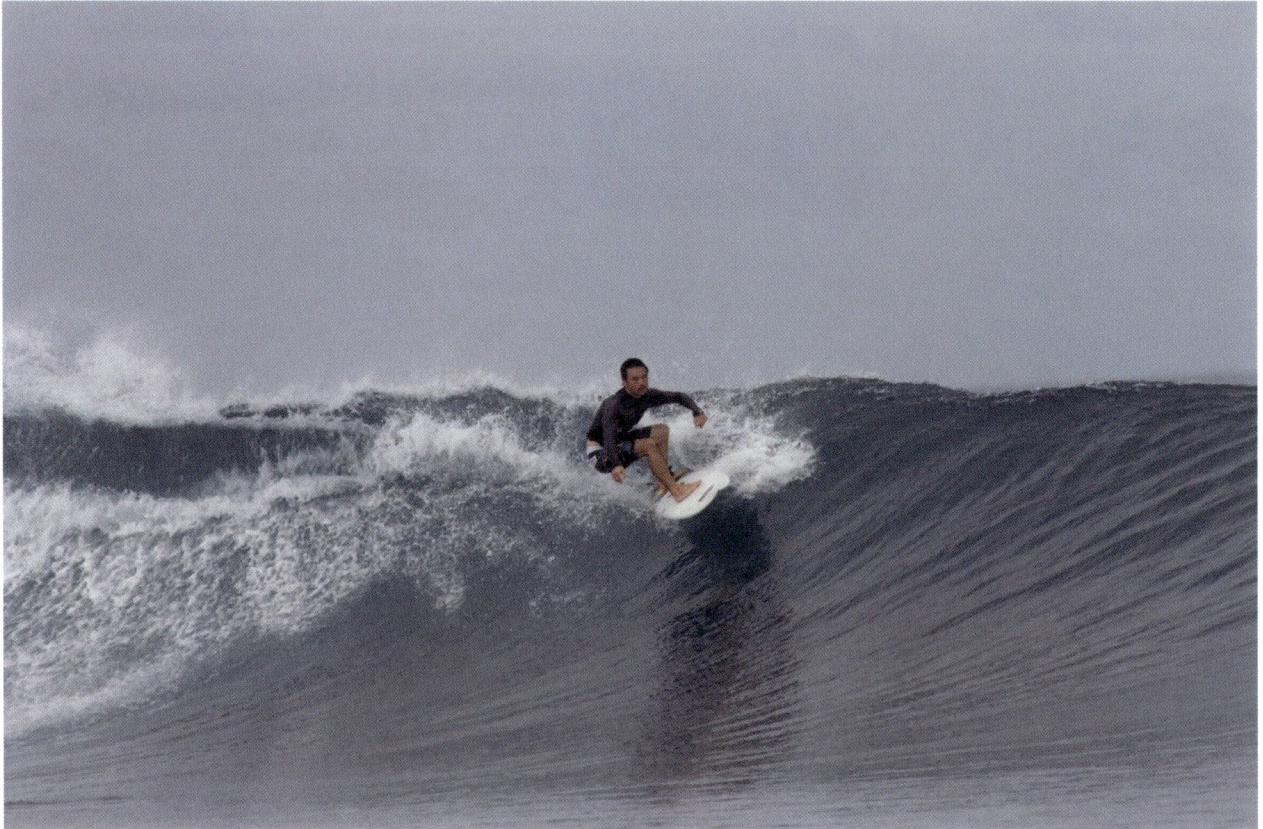

Back in 2016, Pat was surfing one summer day at one of his favorite surf spots. It was the last day of a great week of consistent swell (waves) before a setting off on a week-long surf trip he had planned to Costa Rica. Since he was surfing regularly up until then, he was in my best surfing shape ever.

But, as you may know, that trip never happened. After he took the last wave in, he sprained my ankle getting out of the water.

Not being able to walk for several months he tried to make the best of the situation by establishing my blog - all day I eat like a shark - to share his love for healthy cooking and travel.

He also **read a lot of books.**

Three in particular led him to reassess and gradually change his cooking habits to what they are today: *The Omnivore's Dilemma* **by Michael Pollan,** *The China Study* **and** *Whole* **by T. Colin Campbell.**

If there was any one food that helped him fully make the transition to eating plant-based foods regularly, it was tofu.

So in 2018, he wrote a cookbook on Japanese tofu [Tofu Ryouri -Simple Japanese Tofu Recipes to Cook Healthier at Home](#)**. He believed this cookbook was one way he could help people like you discover new and delicious ways to enjoy tofu, Japanese style!**

For him, [Tofu Ryouri](#) **was a reminder of his progress. This transition wasn't something that happened overnight, but over the course of two years. And it's something he continues to explore and enjoy each week.**

As a second generation Japanese American, it's important for him to share his heritage and empower you to think and cook differently with plant-based Japanese cuisine. More importantly, it's one type of food he believes you can leverage to stay healthy and free of certain chronic diseases.

In his spare time, he continues to challenge himself with new ways of cooking, learning as much as he can and serving as one more bridge to get you across the river to a healthier and longer life.

While there are many bridges that can get you there, he's grateful you've chosen this one. The bridge of tasty, plant-based Japanese food. Perhaps one day, you'll look back 5, 10 or 20 years from now and be grateful you decided to incorporate more plant foods into your life. And maybe it'll bring

back fond memories for you, as you're enjoying each delicious bite or savory scent, helping you revisit or even experience Japan vicariously for the very first time.

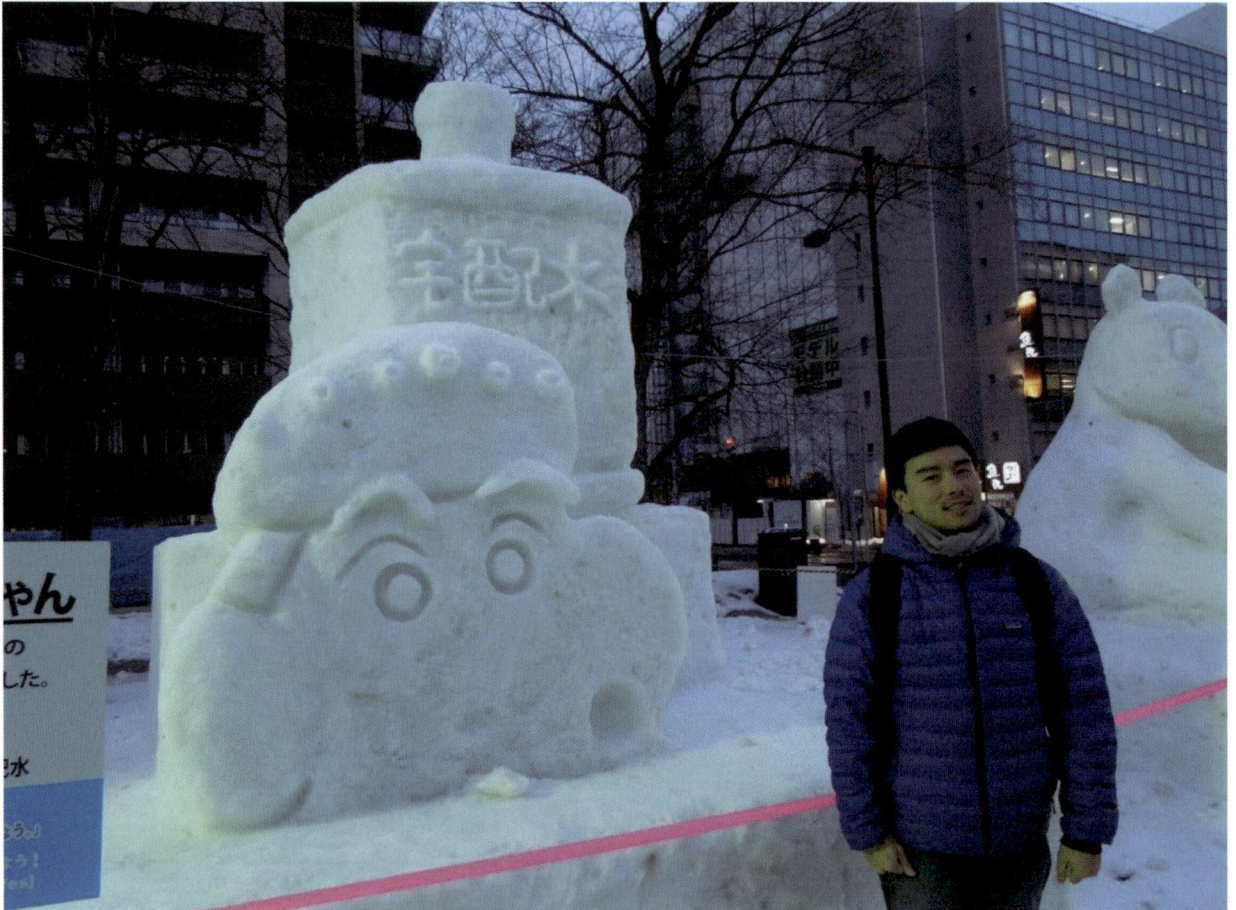

Sapporo Snow Festival, 2013 Sapporo City, Hokkaido, Japan

Do we look alike? That's Crayon Shinchan, my favorite cartoon growing up!

About the Japanese Cooking Club

As you may know, in 2018 Pat began to regularly create cooking videos to share his love of Japanese cuisine via the all day I eat like a shark Youtube channel. He thought it was important to demystify Japanese food through his videos, to make it simple and accessible for home cooks and foodies to recreate in their own kitchen. But one thing was missing...

a community.

He enjoys bringing people of different backgrounds together with food. And he believes that when we come together, we can all learn something from each other. As a result, establishing the Japanese Cooking Club felt like the next natural step.

Through this community and the collective wisdom it can provide, he hopes more people will become informed on the benefits of plant-based foods and also be inspired to take action.

Why?

Because they'll see those around them taking action and enjoying the richly flavored and aromatic aspects of home cooked Japanese food. It's the ripple effect.

The Japanese Cooking Club is one way that he empowers people like you to take more control and responsibility for your health, while also combining two of his passions - food and helping people learn, grow and ensure they live a happy, healthy life! If you're interested in learning more and becoming a member, head to alldayieat.com/go/joinjcc

Printed in Great Britain
by Amazon